WITHDRAWN

Risk Management in Long-Term Care

Andrew D. Weinberg, MD, FACP, has been involved in the long-term care industry for over 15 years and has published many articles dealing with the care of the institutionalized elderly. In the past he has served as a member of the Joint Commission on Accreditation of Healthcare Organization's Professional and Technical Advisory Committee on Long-term Care and as Chairman of the Connecticut State Medical Society's Committee on Geriatrics. He currently serves as the Vice-Chairman of the Committee on Geriatric Medicine of the Massachusetts Medical Society and as the President-elect of the Massachusetts Geriatrics Society (American Geriatrics Society). Dr. Weinberg is the current Medical Director of the Nursing Home Care Unit for the Brockton/West Roxbury VAMC in Brockton, Massachusetts and holds a full-time teaching position in the Division on Aging, Harvard Medical School, Boston. Dr. Weinberg has also served as an expert witness in numerous malpractice cases involving long-term care facilities during the last decade.

Risk Management in Long-Term Care

A Quick Reference Guide

Andrew D. Weinberg, MD, FACP

Springer Publishing Company

Springer Publishing Company, Inc.
536 Broadway
New York, NY 10012-3955

Cover design by Margaret Dunin
Acquisitions Editor: Bill Tucker
Production Editor: Jeanne Libby

98 99 00 01 02/5 4 3 2 1

Weinberg, Andrew David.
    Risk management in long-term care: a quick reference guide /
Andrew Weinberg.
        p.   cm.
    Includes bibliographical references and index.
    ISBN 0-8261-9940-2
    1. Long-term care facilities—Risk management.   I. Title.
RA999.R57W44   1997
362.1'*6'068—dc21   97-25304
                                                                         CIP

Printed in the United States of America

To the nurses, physicians and all healthcare professionals working in the field of long-term care. May we all continue to strive to provide the highest quality care for our seniors.

Contents

Contents

Foreword

Over 1.6 million seniors currently reside in our nation's nursing homes. This number is expected to grow by approximately 25%, to 2 million, by the end of the decade. In recent years, damage awards by juries in nursing home–related negligence cases in the United States have soared. From 1987 to 1994 the average award nearly doubled to $525,000, a figure that excludes additional punitive damages also assessed against homes. In fact, many individual jury awards are now in the millions of dollars, even when the nursing home resident is possibly near the end of his or her life or is severely ill. Currently, there are thousands of cases pending in court, with potential damages approaching $1 billion. Nursing home owners, administrators, and staff need to realize that their first and most important responsibility must be to the residents with whose care they are charged.

Nursing home regulation by federal and state inspectors is not adequate to properly monitor all activities on a frequent basis. However, every year more and more states are considering passing stricter regulations and laws to hold nursing homes legally accountable for the total care of the residents and any untoward effects that may occur during their stay in the facility. Therefore, to ensure that professional care and respect are given to all residents at all times, nursing homes must become the leaders in providing quality care.

Dr. Andrew Weinberg's *Risk Management and Long-Term Care: A Quick Reference Guide* is clearly the most practical, effective, and thorough risk management tool available to long-term care institutions to address these critical issues. This publication covers the prevention of potential legal action as well as the appropriate responses when such claims arise. Dr. Weinberg identifies potential problem areas and gives easy-to-understand tips on how to avoid liability while improving the delivery of care. His overall philosophy of risk management is predicated on promoting and enhancing the quality of resident life in long-term care settings.

Risk Management and Long-Term Care offers numerous case examples, specific suggestions, and recommended policies and procedures to follow in providing quality care and thereby manage risk. Careful adherence to Dr. Weinberg's logical approach will markedly reduce liability for long-term care institutions and provide for a happier and healthier resident population. This book is a "must read" for anyone involved with long-term care.

James L. Wilkes II, Esq.
October 1996

James L. Wilkes II is a founding partner of Wilkes & McHugh, PA, of Tampa, Florida. He is a frequent lecturer across the country on nursing home issues and has testified on nursing home resident neglect and abuse before the Florida State Legislature. Mr. Wilkes was chairman of the Nursing Home Litigation Strike Force of the Academy of Florida Trial Lawyers and a past member of the board of directors of the Academy of Florida Trial Lawyers, and is a member of the Florida Bar Association, the American Bar Association, and the American Institute of Medical Law. Mr. Wilkes has had extensive experience in civil trial practice involving complex medical litigation and is one of the most successful plaintiff attorneys in nursing home and medical malpractice litigation. He is a well-known national advocate for improvement in delivery of care in the long-term-care setting.

1

Introduction and Overview

Risk management, simply defined, is the provision of quality care by the identification of potential and actual problems with subsequent formulation of solutions to alleviate these problems. Risk management should be thought of as a *continuum* of evaluation, treatment and on-going monitoring of conditions in a nursing facility. With changes that are constantly occurring in the health care milieu effecting the facility's mission, staffing patterns, number of beds or types of service provided, there may need to be modifications of any risk management program in place. An effective risk management program also requires the identification of high-risk areas and procedures and the implementation of corrective or preventive actions throughout a facility in an organized fashion.

Many long-term care facilities provide a variety of nursing, medical, recreational, and rehabilitative services to their residents, and the potential for injury tends to be significant in such a frail, older population. Areas for concern include an understanding of the entire spectrum of responsibilities of the administrative, medical, and nursing staff that are required under the Omnibus Budget Reconciliation Act (OBRA), as well as ongoing monitoring of identified areas of potential risk in the resident population of the nursing home. It should be recognized that teamwork is critical in any successful risk management program. Although it is impossible to prevent all risk, effective management strategies can reduce its occurrence and minimize injury to residents while improving the quality of care being delivered.

Overall, litigation involving nursing homes remains relatively rare, compared to the number of malpractice suits filed against hospitals and private physicians. Nonetheless, in several states there have been annual increases in the per-bed malpractice premium of up to 25%.[1] Moreover, there appears to be potential for a significant increase in lawsuits as long-term care (LTC) facilities venture into the subacute market and provide increased services such as peritoneal dialysis and intravenous therapy for their residents. Furthermore, with the coming increase in prospective payment systems, which may result in the admission of seriously ill patients directly to LTC facilities, the incidence of malpractice suits against nursing homes based on poor or substandard care may increase.

1

This book is intended to serve as a guide not only for nursing home administrators, directors of nursing, and medical directors, but for all attending physicians, staff nurses, nurse practitioners, and physician assistants motivated to provide quality care to the residents for whom they are responsible. Risk management should be thought of as a continuum of evaluation, treatment, and ongoing monitoring of conditions in a nursing facility. With changes that are constantly occurring in the health care milieu affecting the facility's mission, staffing patterns, number of beds, or types of services provided, there may need to be modifications of any risk management program in place.

The methods described in this book will allow your facility to create a highly effective risk management program to address the most common concerns involved in the delivery of care that may arise in a nursing home setting. Readers should come away with a better understanding of how to avoid injuries among residents and to use quality improvement techniques as a morale booster. The recommendations given are practical and can be implemented easily in any long-term care facility. Good risk management needs to involve all staff members in identifying potential danger areas to both residents and staff and in formulating a plan of corrective action.

Like lawsuits, not all injuries and accidents can be prevented. However, by identifying the causative factors of any untoward events and assembling an intervention strategy to prevent repetition of an incident, overall quality of care will improve. Improving communication, not only with family members but with the staff, can go a long way in minimizing confusion and conflicting feelings and will allow any complaints or disputes to be resolved without the input from attorneys. Finally, any facility policies that are in place must be practical enough to be carried out by the staff with currently available resources and must be adhered to by all parties.

ACKNOWLEDGMENT. The author wishes to thank Jean K. Pals, RN, C, BSN, for her helpful suggestions in the preparation of this book.

REFERENCES

1. Fraser. Nursing home civil litigation. *Nursing Home Med.* 1995; 3:79–82.

2

Approach to Risk Management in the Long-Term Care Setting

Although risk management in-servicing of LTC staff is increasing across the country, few facilities have formal programs in place. Risk management must ideally involve all disciplines working in a facility, including the medical director, staff physicians, and other consultants.[1,2]

Effective risk management also requires a 24-hour-a-day, 7-days-a-week commitment on the part of staff and administration, with the flexibility to effectively respond to all identified problems and high-risk procedures. Key areas that need to be addressed include:

1. *New admissions.* Many times, residents being admitted to a facility for the first time come with little information. Transfer forms may have scanty, missing, or even inaccurate information, especially as it relates to current medications, intravenous therapy, or consultant recommendations that were made in the hospital. The admissions coordinator should make every effort to obtain as much medical information as possible about a prospective resident *prior* to admission. Many lawsuits have resulted from error in medication administration, treatments, diet, and hydration that were due to confusion on the part of the receiving facility regarding what was actually being done for the resident in the previous health care setting. If the nursing staff has any doubts regarding a treatment or medication for a new admission, call the referring facility immediately. Calling the attending physician at the nursing home may not be as helpful as contacting the referring facility since many times the nursing home attending physician may not have known the resident prior to this admission. Never assume the transfer form is totally complete. Family members consulted about recent hospital-related events may prove a valuable source of information regarding current treatments, diet, and other required interventions.

2. *Education.* In-servicing nursing assistants and licensed staff on all areas of potential injury to residents, staff, and visitors in the nursing home setting is vital. Repetition of these programs must be dictated by ongoing clinical needs and staff turnover rates.

3. *Documentation.* Proper and complete documentation by all staff members and attending physicians is another critical issue. For legal purposes, if it is not documented in the resident's record, it is assumed that the medication or treatment was not given or done. Care plans need to be comprehensive and address each issue in detail.

4. *Critical incident reports.* Use these reports to detect and document trends and hazardous areas where improvement is indicated.

5. *Communication.* Always strive to maintain effective two-way communication and a cooperative attitude with family members. Also, maintain good channels of communication with staff members and listen to their complaints and suggestions.

It is generally believed that the staff of any LTC facility will only take risk management programs seriously to the extent to which they perceive the administration is supporting the program. Therefore, the administration must be actively involved with the design, implementation, monitoring of, and compliance with all risk management endeavors in their facility.

The primary areas of citations of LTC facilities by the Health Care Financing Administration usually involve deficiencies in

- Storage and distribution of food under sanitary conditions
- Comprehensive resident care plans
- Comprehensive assessment of residents' needs based on minimum data set
- Safety
- Housekeeping and maintenance services to maintain sanitary interior

Proponents of continuous quality improvement (CQI) programs propose that redesigning systems, protocols, and procedures to meet clinical needs is the primary way to improve care within a facility, rather than identifying and punishing those deemed "at fault" in any one specific incident. Many advocate the integration of risk management and CQI programs within a facility as an ideal method of improving care and minimizing risk.[3]

The formation of a risk management team can help facilitate the organization and implementation of a facility's program. This team should meet on a regular basis and focus on areas that have high-risk potential (see Table 2.1). This team could also be charged with regularly reviewing all facility policies and protocols and recommending changes as needed. Their work should interact with and complement the CQI program of a facility as much as possible.

TABLE 2.1   Areas of High-Risk Potential in a Long-Term Care
Facility

- Allergic reactions to medications and staff-response protocols
- Fall-related injuries
- Loss (theft) or destruction of resident property
- Medical illness/failure to diagnosis or treat properly
- Medication errors
- Pressure ulcers: monitoring, evaluation, and treatment issues
- Resident-to-resident assaults
- Resident-to-staff assaults
- Resident abuse by staff
- Subacute unit medical/staff coverage issues
- Unclear or unfair admission and discharge policies
- Violation of residents' rights
- Wandering/elopement-related injuries (e.g., fractures and other trauma, hypothermia, death)

SUBACUTE UNITS

With the significant increase in the formation of subacute units within LTC facilities in the past few years, it is crucial that adequate staffing and responsible medical coverage be available 7 days a week, not just on day shifts Monday through Friday. With a growing number of admissions coming on late Friday afternoon or the weekend, the usual tendency to schedule less staff on weekends, nights, and holidays seen in many LTC facilities must be avoided at all costs. Contact the designated attending physician as soon as possible so he or she is informed of the scheduled admission. Although many facilities may not be aware when a resident is coming for admission until the last moment, it is vitally important that there be an admitting physician available to care for the new admission and physically examine him or her within 48 hours (or sooner, if required by state or facility policy). If physician coverage is inadequate over the weekends and holidays per nursing staff's report, then the medical director should be asked to investigate this complaint as soon as possible and report back to the administration on possible solutions. The potential scope of duties of the medical director as they relate to subacute units has been described in detail elsewhere.[4]

Because these units often manage intravenous and central lines in their residents, the director of nursing should ascertain that the training level of assigned staff on all shifts is adequate to care for the lines being used. Emergency phone numbers of supervisory staff should be prominently posted throughout the unit, and the staff should be actively encouraged to use them whenever needed. The director of nursing, the medical director, and other crucial staff members (e.g., physical therapists) should also review all potential subacute admissions for appropriateness and to ensure the facility will have properly trained staff to administer the required treatments before agreeing to the admission.

When a new licensed staff member is hired, proper training and documentation of skills should be completed prior to letting that individual work unsupervised on any subacute unit. Records of training received by all staff members should be stored in a central location, and retraining for any specialized procedures should be given on a regular basis. Contingency plans for resignations, illnesses and vacations should be made in advance and publicized to all supervisors to avoid having untrained staff working in a subacute unit.

While subacute units allow many LTC facilities to offer advanced levels of care for residents with the benefit of potentially increased reimbursement, the risks of caring for unstable or potentially unstable residents in a nonhospital setting can present the possibility of untoward results for the residents if proper planning, organization, and supervision are not employed.

The techniques that are presented in this book are designed to heighten the awareness of nursing home administrators, directors of nursing, medical directors, and staff members in the provision of improved quality care to their residents. The recommendations, however, must be reviewed and modified, updated as clinical needs dictate. All recommendations given can be implemented without massive increases in expenditures by the facility or major changes in current operational methods. However, the active commitment and participation of the staff, physicians, consultants, and administration are critical if any risk management program is to succeed in its primary mission: providing quality care.

REFERENCES

1. Allen JE. Effective risk management in long-term care. *J of Long-Term Care Admin.* 1991; 19:43–46, 49.
2. Kapp MD. Preventing malpractice in long-term care: Strategies for risk management. New York: Springer Publishing Co., 1987.
3. Micheletti J, Shlala T. Integrating risk management and quality assurance programs. *Contemporary LTC.* 1988; 11:79–83.
4. Dimant J. The role of the medical director in subacute care. *Nurs Home Med.* 1995; 3:115–121.

10 Tips From This Chapter

1. Quality control and delivery of quality care remain the primary focus of good risk management.
2. Education of all staff on high-risk clinical issues is critical. Repeat programs based on need and staff turnover.
3. To be effective, any risk management program must be comprehensive, organized, and supported by staff and administration. Listen carefully to staff members regarding suggested improvements to current operating procedures and facility policies, and regularly seek their input.
4. Consider the creation of a risk management team to facilitate the identification and resolution of high-risk areas and procedures.
5. Do not assume information on transfer forms from an acute care hospital is complete. Always investigate any areas where there is confusion or possible omission of required treatments and medications.
6. LTC facilities must avoid the tendency to schedule fewer staff members on weekends, nights, and holidays in subacute units.
7. Emergency phone numbers of supervisory staff should be prominently posted throughout the unit, and staff members should be actively encouraged to use them whenever needed.
8. Review all potential subacute admissions for appropriateness and the ability to provide required services.
9. Records of training received by staff members for any specialized procedures should be stored in a central location and retraining given on a regular basis to maintain clinical competency.
10. Contingency plans for resignations, illnesses, and vacations should be made in advance and publicized to all supervisors to avoid having untrained staff working in a subacute unit.

3

Pressure Ulcers

Pressure ulcers, while making up less than 10% of all claims, constitute the vast majority of economic loss for negligence suits filed against nursing homes and physicians. Although the treatment of pressure ulcers has advanced tremendously in the last decade, the only way to guarantee good results is to prevent their occurrence, whenever possible, through the use of aggressive prevention programs.[1,2,3,4] The estimated cost for treating a single pressure ulcer can range from $5,000 to $40,000 or even higher, and the prevalence of pressure ulcers in long-term care populations may range from 2.4% to 23%.[4] Severely infected pressure ulcers can lead to sepsis and death, and the estimated mortality in those residents with bacteremia and pressure ulcers has been associated with a mortality rate of 50%.[5]

The Agency for Health Care Policy and Research has released research-based methods for appropriately treating pressure ulcers.[1] These treatment guidelines stress that intervention for at-risk long-term care residents needs to be implemented early. The guidelines should be the basis for any treatment plan involving skin integrity. Pressure ulcers generally form over bony prominences and are graded according to the degree of tissue damage present. The staging system can be summarized as follows[1]:

Stage I: Nonblanchable erythema of intact skin.

Stage II: Partial-thickness skin loss that involves the epidermis and/or dermis. This type of pressure ulcer is superficial and can present as a blister, abrasion, or shallow crater.

Stage III: Full-thickness skin loss involving significant damage or necrosis of subcutaneous tissue that may extend down to, but not through, the underlying fascia. This type of pressure ulcer may present clinically as a deep crater with or without undermining of adjacent tissue.

Stage IV: Full-thickness skin loss involving extensive destruction, tissue necrosis, or damage to muscle, bone, or supporting structures. Undermining and sinus tracts may also be associated with this stage.

It is important to emphasize that when eschar is present, a pressure ulcer cannot be accurately graded. Such an ulcer may require frequent reassessment to ensure that misgrading does not occur. Eschar removal may be needed before accurate grading can be accomplished.

In residents wearing certain orthopedic devices, the early detection of pressure ulcers may be extremely difficult and extra monitoring may be required. All residents admitted with any prosthetic device or cast should be considered at very high risk for pressure ulcer development. Initial nursing care plans should stress the monitoring of these sites on a regular basis.

All treatment programs for pressure ulcers should comprise at least the following:

1. Initial assessment of all residents for potential of skin breakdown. If it is determined that a resident is at high risk for pressure ulcer development, this potential problem needs to be addressed in the initial nursing care plan.
2. Documentation of all pressure ulcers for location, size (length, width, and depth), stage, the presence of any sinus tracts, undermining, tunneling, exudate, and necrotic tissue. Additionally, the presence or absence of granulation tissue and epithelialization should be noted.
3. Formulation of a plan of care involving the entire treatment team, including the attending physician.
4. Assessment of any contributing medical, nutritional, or hydration problems. Nutritional assessment should follow the guidelines as defined by the Nutrition Screening Initiative.
5. Reassessment of all pressure ulcers on a regular basis.
6. Establishment of reasonable treatment goals based on the resident's overall health and his or her wishes. If the resident is not competent, the legal next of kin should be consulted.
7. Inclusion of consultative assistance (e.g., surgical consult for debridement intervention) when conservative treatment methods fail to improve the pressure ulcer within a specified time frame.

Although different support surfaces exist for the resident with pressure ulcers (e.g., air-fluidized, low air loss, static flotation, and foam or alternating-air beds), the primary consideration for selecting the ideal surface is the therapeutic benefit associated with the product. Support surfaces are only one part of a comprehensive treatment plan. If healing is not occurring, evaluate the entire treatment plan and not just the support surface being used. If a consultant recommends the use of a specific support surface, it is critical to either follow the recommendation or document in the chart the reason that the recommendation is not being implemented at this time.

While it is well known that certain characteristics of long-term care residents increase their propensity for pressure ulcer development (e.g., physical disabilities, immobility, psychiatric problems, incontinence, anemia, malnutrition, chronic medical illness, and prosthetic devices), the legal argument seen in all malpractice/negligence suits is that pressure ulcers are preventable and, if not preventable, are always treatable. The fact that a particular resident was admitted with a Stage III or Stage IV pressure ulcer is, by itself, a poor defense for why it stayed that way or worsened. Color photographs of pressure ulcers taken at the time of admission, while helpful in documenting the presence and staging of these ulcers when first encountered by the staff of a facility, does not reduce the obligation to prevent their progression. For this reason, it is imperative that the director of nursing and the medical director of each facility be fully aware and review the appropriateness of any admission being considered to determine if proper resources are present to treat any preexisting pressure ulcer.

Federal OBRA regulations state[6]:

Based on the comprehensive assessment of a resident, the facility must ensure that: (1) a resident who enters a facility without pressure sores does not develop pressure sores unless the individual's clinical condition demonstrates that they were unavoidable; and (2) a resident having pressure sores receives the necessary treatment and services to promote healing, prevent infection, and prevent new sores from developing.

The resident assessment instrument in the minimum data set and the resident assessment protocols are required to be completed on each nursing home resident in your facility. This information should be used by your skin care team to help identify at-risk residents for pressure ulcer development.

Risk management programs looking at pressure ulcer prevention should identify on admission all residents having the following characteristics:

- immobility of any type
- diabetes mellitus
- significant peripheral vascular disease
- paraplegia or quadriplegia
- amputation
- severe pulmonary obstructive disease
- chronic bowel or urinary incontinence
- significant malnutrition or dehydration
- casts of any type
- chronic or end-stage liver or renal disease
- terminal cancer
- extended time that the head of the bed must be elevated due to medical necessity

It is critical to point out that when you have an order to "turn resident every 2 hours," legally you must turn and document that turn *every* 2 hours. A medical record that shows significant gaps in documentation will be presumed to indicate that the turning was not done. Because Stage I or Stage II pressure ulcers can develop within approximately 2 hours, it is imperative that if you are going to provide such treatments to your residents, you should ensure that all shifts have adequate staffing. Failure to regularly reposition residents as ordered is very often cited in allegations of negligent care, so repositioning needs to be documented carefully on all shifts. Additionally, failure to provide adequate staffing is a common plaintiff theme and one that is hard to refute. Juries have little sympathy for a facility's staffing problems. If you cannot provide adequate staffing for a care-intensive resident, you should either not accept that resident for admission or work on transferring him or her to another facility that will agree to provide this required level of care. Documentation of appropriate training of personnel involved in turning and repositioning of residents is also important.

Your facility's intervention plan should be detailed and assigned to one individual or a number of highly committed and organized individuals to assess and track pressure ulcers among your resident population. Assessment tools, flow sheets, and prevention and treatment protocols should be developed to deal with the different stages of pressure ulcers, and these protocols and any associated nursing policies should be in-serviced to all nursing assistants and licensed personnel. This training is important for all staff and should be carefully documented. Regular offerings of this training are also imperative. Early recognition of Stage I pressure ulcers remains the chief way of lowering the cost of services and improving quality of care for at-risk residents.

The use of oral zinc and ascorbic acid in the treatment of pressure ulcers has been advocated in some published reports,[7] but their routine use is not universally recognized. The routine use of topical antibiotics and antiseptics is also quite controversial. Although the use of antibiotics and antiseptics can help decrease bacterial counts and potentially promote healing, povidone-iodine, acetic acid, and hydrogen peroxide can be cytotoxic and damage granulation tissue. Other agents, such as triple antibiotics and silver sulfadiazine, may also be indicated at times to reduce purulent drainage or foul odor that can be present in certain pressure ulcers.[1] The use of all such agents should be thoroughly discussed with the attending physician based on each resident's clinical needs.

Since most pressure ulcers should show healing in 2 to 4 weeks, failure to note such healing is a clear indication to reevaluate your treatment plan and to determine if all elements have been followed by the staff. Documentation of pressure ulcer healing or progression is critical and should include, at minimum, the following:

- date and time of exam
- stage of ulcer and any change since last exam
- preventive measures being undertaken
- nutritional and hydration status of resident
- treatments currently being administered

If there are gaps in the treatment record, these may be used to indicate that "no care at all" was being given, which may be patently untrue. However, as stated before, if staff members fail to document treatments, such treatments are assumed, for legal purposes, not to have been done. An effort should be made to audit charts regularly to look for gaps in documentation, and appropriate follow-up of these identified areas should be pursued. All concurrent medical problems, including dehydration and malnourishment, need to be addressed in the care plan with follow-through by the staff. Because medical illnesses can greatly accelerate the progression of a pressure ulcer or impede its healing, these problems must be aggressively pursued and resolved to maximize the healing process.

Regarding the use of camera documentation of pressure ulcers, some consultants and legal advisors have actually told nursing home administrators never to photograph pressure ulcers, since they can be used against the facility in a lawsuit. However, the proper photographing and sequential documentation of healing ulcers or fully healed ulcers can be very helpful in defending against any charges of negligence. Photographs can serve as an objective yardstick to the effectiveness of your care plan in promoting the healing of the pressure ulcers and allow the improvement to be documented on a regular basis for the skin care team. Whether or not photographs are used in any facility depends on the particular needs for such documentation. Regardless of whether photographs are taken, good nursing assessment notes are required to document the treatment and status of all pressure ulcers present in a facility.

In summary, although pressure ulcers are time consuming and potentially expensive to treat, an organized and systematic approach can make the prevention and treatment of pressure ulcers an attainable goal.

REFERENCES

1. Bergstrom N, Bennett MA, Carlson CE, et al. *Pressure Ulcer Treatment.* Clinical Practice Guideline. Quick Reference Guide for Clinicians, No. 15. Rockville, MD: U.S. Department of Health and Human Services, Public Health Service, Agency for Health Care Policy and Research. AHCPR Pub. No. 95-0653, December 1994.
2. Harbit MD. Computer identification of patients at risk for skin breakdown. *Clin Nurse Specialist.* 1996; 10(3):125–127.
3. Kemp MG, Krouskop TA. Pressure ulcers: Reducing the incidence and severity by managing pressure. *J Gerontol Nurs.* 1994; 20(9):27–34.
4. National Pressure Ulcer Advisory Panel (NPUAP). Pressure ulcers prevalence, cost and risk assessment: Consensus development conference statement. *Decubitus.* 1989: May 2(2):24–28.

5. Smith, DM. Pressure ulcers in the nursing home. *Ann Intern Med.* 1995; 123:433–442.
6. Omnibus Budget Reconciliation Acts (OBRA) of 1987, 1989, and 1990. Health Care Financing Administration, as published in the *Federal Register,* September 26, 1991 and March 6, 1992 and Interpretive Guidelines of April 1, 1992.
7. Sih R. Pressure ulcers in the nursing home. *Nurs Home Med.* 1996; 4:193–198.

---

10 Tips From This Chapter

1. Monitor the incidence and prevalence of pressure ulcers on a regular basis.
2. Early identification of Stage I pressure ulcers is key to preventing progression.
3. Involve the attending physician in all treatment decisions and keep him or her informed of any progression of a pressure ulcer.
4. Identify potential stressors for all residents (e.g., prosthesis pressure) and develop interventions to reduce or eliminate such stressors.
5. Incorporate continuous quality improvement monitoring of pressure ulcer management as a major aspect of nursing home care. Monitor for recurrence in all residents with documented pressure ulcers.
6. Consider forming a skin care team to follow all pressure ulcers in a facility and to coordinate treatment. This team should be interdisciplinary in membership.
7. Have the director of nursing and the medical director review all potential admissions with known Stage III or Stage IV pressure ulcers to ascertain whether the facility has the staffing and expertise to handle this level of ulcer.
8. Develop and offer on a regular basis educational programs regarding the facility's approach to the prevention, identification, and treatment of pressure ulcers. Update educational materials presented as required.
9. Always involve the family and resident, whenever possible, in the prevention and treatment of pressure ulcers.
10. Assess nutritional and hydrational needs of all residents at risk for or with the presence of pressure ulcers.

4

Issues Related to Polypharmacy and Medication Use

Medication use is high among residents of long-term care facilities. High utilization often lends itself to potential medication errors or the ongoing problem of polypharmacy in this population. With more acutely ill residents being transferred from acute care hospitals into long-term care facilities, there are often times when complicated medication orders, including intravenous (IV) drugs, accompany these new admissions.

In many cases, the prescribing of newer, more expensive medications to replace older ones with proven safety records does not necessarily represent an improvement in overall pharmacological therapy for the older person. Overall, there are some basic questions that need to be asked before nursing staff should request any centrally acting medication that can affect behavior:

1. What are the target symptoms the medication is being requested to control? Are they, in fact, treatable with medication?
2. Have nonpharmacological alternatives been tried? (Nonpharmacological methods to treat nonbehavioral-related problems should be utilized whenever possible.)
3. Would discontinuing a current medication relieve some of the existing symptoms?
4. By what criteria will the effects of the new medication therapy be assessed?

Psychiatric and behavioral concerns constitute the primary reasons the nursing staff requests new medication orders from attending physicians. It has been estimated that 90% of nursing home residents may exhibit the following noncognitive behavioral problems at some time.[1] These target symptoms most often include:

- screaming
- sleep-related problems
- aggressive/agitated behavior

Traditional neuroleptics have been used for decades as primary therapy for many of these symptoms. However, serious side effects can result, including tardive dyskinesia, sedation, extrapyramidal symptoms, increased falls, and confusion. Subsequent problems can also include the development of dehydration through decreased fluid intake. Physiological changes in metabolism occur as one gets older, and this fact can increase the risk of drug reactions[2,3] and necessitate more extensive management in the older person.[4,5] The use of centrally-acting medications, such as neuroleptics and benzodiazepines, can also increase the risk for hip fracture.[6,7]

Overall, good data on the toxicity and efficacy of pharmacotherapeutic options for use in residents of nursing homes are limited and the exact relationship between risks and benefits of all medication use in this population must be carefully scrutinized by the prescribing physician.[8]

Medication-related problems can be divided into three major areas:

1. incorrect/inappropriate dosage ordered
2. failure to note a previously documented drug allergy
3. nursing administration error

Communication errors, transcription errors, and failure to notify the attending physician of medication-related problems are also important factors in this area. On admission to a nursing home facility, it is important to verify with the referring facility which of the daily ordered medications have been given and to ensure that the vendor pharmacy can deliver all required medications in a timely fashion to allow the prescribed medication regimen to be administered.

It is also important that a clinical reason for each ordered medication be known and documented. Continuing a medicine just because "the resident was sent out of the hospital on it" is using poor judgment. However, multiple medications should not be discontinued simultaneously. In general, the discontinuation or reduction in dose of one medication at a time is usually the best approach to allow for the individual response to the change to be properly assessed. If there is any doubt about the need for or the dose of a particular medication, call the referring facility and ask to speak with the attending physician to clarify any pertinent issues.

Regular in-services should be held on proper charting of medications, narcotic box procedures, and security, along with potential side effects and clinical actions of commonly prescribed medications. Also, for those facilities with IV programs, proper initial training and retraining on a regular basis needs to be available for all staff members working with IV fluids and medications. Nurses should be aware of their obligation to call the medical director on any medication-related problem if the primary attending or covering physician cannot be reached in a timely manner. All allergic-type or serious side effects of a medication need to discussed with the attending physician immediately. Most severe allergic reactions should be treated in an acute care setting until stabilized. Any change in mental status of a resident may be related to a potential medication side effect.

Consulting pharmacists can be helpful to a facility in identifying medication-related issues for the staff and training/implementing intervention techniques. These areas include:

- conducting in-services on common drug interactions and side effects of commonly prescribed medications
- reviewing current medication policies for the facility
- reviewing and critiquing medication errors for any possible patterns
- providing narcotic security
- helping staff to identify prn or other routine medications that could potentially be discontinued
- working with staff/attending physicians to decrease the dosage or discontinue neuropharmacologically active agents on a regular basis
- working with the attending physician to minimize the total number of medications prescribed while allowing the desired clinical benefit to be realized

The medical director and other attending physician staff may be helpful in addressing the above issues. The in-service coordinator of a facility should approach these individuals to see if they would participate in educating the staff on a particular pharmacological issue in which they themselves feel well versed. Nursing supervisors should avoid scheduling different nurses on the same shift to distribute medications to minimize the possibility of administration errors. If at all possible, avoid having medication nurses work double-shifts as tiredness can increase the frequency of medication errors.

Below is a case study that illustrates how to avoid typical medication-related problems.

CASE STUDY

On Wednesday morning Dr. Williams, the attending physician for several residents at Willow Manor Nursing Home, is notified by the nursing staff of the East wing that a long-term care resident, with a history of probable Alzheimer's disease, is becoming more agitated in the late afternoons. This has been occurring since he had a new roommate assigned to his room. The nursing staff has noticed this behavior in the past but had always been able to manage these episodes using cue-ing and other nonpharmacological techniques. During the last two weeks the sit-uation, according to the nursing staff, has become unmanageable. The nurses are requesting that a telephone order for Haldol be given to help "calm" the resident.

After reviewing with the staff over the telephone any clinical symptoms that might indicate acute medical illness, Dr. Williams gives an order for Haldol 0.5 mg by mouth 3 times a day. The next Saturday a staff member calls Dr. Williams's covering physician, Dr. Bennett, again stating the resident is even more restless despite the regular use of Haldol during the preceding week. The nurse is request-ing an increase in the Haldol order to help control this escalating restlessness. Dr. Bennett gives an order to increase the Haldol to 1 mg 3 times a day. Two days later, staff members note the resident to be extremely restless, unable to sit still for even a few minutes, and refusing all personal care and food. The attending physician is called to obtain an order to transfer the resident to an acute psychiatric facility for emergency evaluation.

Comments

A common theme in long-term care geriatrics is that an adverse drug effect can mimic almost any clinical syndrome. This case study follows the pattern of a res-ident most likely experiencing akathisia, an extrapyramidal side effect of neu-roleptic therapy. Akathisia is a common drug-induced symptom in older people and can resemble agitation. It is best defined as motor restlessness with a com-pulsion to continuously move. Giving increased doses of a neuroleptic only serves to increase the symptoms.

Initial therapy for these symptoms would be to decrease the dose of the offend-ing neuroleptic and reassess the behavior. Before initiating any neuroleptic med-ication, it is advisable that the attending physician examine the resident and order any laboratory testing that could be indicated to rule out acute medical problems as the cause of the change in behavior. Additionally, before starting any specific drug therapy, it is critical to identify the target behavior to be treated and to define the goals of therapy. Always start with the lowest possible dose and prescribe only short courses of treatment with continued reevaluation of the clinical status. Staff should monitor the resident closely for the development of possible side effects, which include decreased appetite and fluid intake, sedation, confusion, and increased risk for falling. It is very important that all medication use be reviewed frequently for appropriateness of dose and specific clinical indications.

Medication-related problems can be minimized with an organized and system-atic approach to the storage, documentation, and administration of medications within the nursing home. In-service educational sessions on common medication-related errors should be presented on a regular basis to help heighten the aware-ness among nursing staff of potential areas of concern.

REFERENCES

1. Goldberg RJ, Goldberg, J. Antipsychotics for dementia-related behavioral disturbances in elderly institutionalized patients. *Nursing Home Med.* 1996; 4:201–206.
2. Gurwitz J, Avorn J. The ambiguous relation between aging and adverse drug reactions. *Ann Int Med.* 1991; 114:956–966.
3. Nolan L, O'Malley K. Prescribing for the elderly. Part I: Sensitivity of the elderly to adverse drug reactions. *J Am Geriatr Soc.* 1988; 36:142–149.
4. Montamat SC, Cusack BJ, Vestal RE. Management of drug therapy in the elderly. *NEJM.* 1989; 321:303–309.
5. Gurwitz JH, Soumerai SB, Avorn J. Improving medication prescribing and utilization in the nursing home. *J Am Geriatr Soc.* 1990; 38:542–552.
6. Ray WA, Griffin MR, Schaffmer W, et al. Psychotropic drug use and the risk of hip fracture. *NEJM.* 1987; 316:363–369.
7. Ray WA, Griffin MR, Downey W. Benzodiazepines of long and short elimination half-life and the risk of hip fracture. *JAMA.* 1989; 262:3303–3307.
8. Avon J, Gurwitz JH. Drug use in the nursing home. *Ann Intern Med.* 1995; 123:195–204.

10 Tips From This Chapter

1. Always identify the clinical reason for each medication being prescribed. If in doubt, call the referring facility.
2. Ensure that the vendor pharmacy is able to make timely deliveries of medications for new admissions to prevent administration-time-related incidents.
3. Supervise In-service nurses regularly on proper administration and charting of all medications, including narcotic procedures.
4. When the primary attending physician of record is not reachable, the medical director of the facility should be contacted for any serious medication-related incidents.
5. Consultant pharmacists should be contacted to help identify any possible patterns to the medication errors and to help formulate interventions to ensure proper administration of medications.
6. Nursing staff should be encouraged to identify "prn" or routine medications no longer clinically indicated for a particular resident and to notify the attending physician of these recommendations.
7. In-service education should be conducted on a regular basis regarding the understanding of drug interactions in the older person and common medication side effects. Nurses involved with the facility's IV program should also be regularly retrained on protocols and procedures.
8. In conjunction with the attending physician, attempt the reduction or discontinuation of neuropharmacological agents on a regular basis with the aim of minimizing the utilization of such medications.
9. The attending physician should be notified immediately about all serious medication-related reactions.
10. Staff should be encouraged to employ nonpharmacological interventions whenever possible to control behavioral-related or insomnia-type problems.

5

Physical Restraints and Neuropsychoactive Medication Use

Risk management continues to dominate any discussion on the issue of physical restraints and the administration of major and minor tranquilizers (neuropsychoactive medications). This chapter will highlight the important concerns that long-term care facilities face when developing policies and procedures covering these two important topics.

RESTRAINTS

Restraints are defined as any devices or objects that the individual cannot easily remove and that restrict freedom of movement or normal access to his or her body. Examples include, but are not limited to, belts, vest restraints, shoulder harnesses, geriatric chairs with tray tables, pelvic/arm/leg restraints, very tightly tucked bedsheets, and wheelchair safety bars that prevent a resident from rising out of the chair. Electronic wristbands or other devices that trigger alarms are not considered restraints, but a resident has the right, if competent, to refuse to wear such devices. Any supportive device that a resident can easily remove is also not considered a restraint. Obviously, restraints should never be used as a form of discipline or for staff convenience. They are not innocuous devices and have caused resident deaths when used incorrectly or not adequately monitored.[1,2]

Full bed rails are considered restraints if they prevent a resident's egress from the bed. Appropriately signed consent forms are needed if they are used. Inappropriately used bed rails have also caused injury and death to significant numbers of nursing home residents. Alternatives to the use of bed rails should be considered and include:

1. Use of an overbed trapeze to increase resident mobility and ability to position oneself in bed

2. Frequent nighttime monitoring of residents by staff
3. Beds placed close to the floor
4. Residents on a frequent toileting program at night
5. Electronic devices used as an adjunct tool to detect when residents arise from their beds
6. Encouragement of residents to call the staff for help when attempting to get out of their beds

Concerns regarding the use of physical restraints are summarized in Table 5.1. Research appears to support the notion that the use of restraints does not, in fact, reduce the incidence of serious fall-related injuries. They should also never be used as a means of controlling wandering or possible elopement. Many legal and ethical issues have arisen when restraints are used without obtaining informed consent, if used or monitored inappropriately, or if applied when less restrictive alternatives have not been attempted.[3-6] All restraint policies need to incorporate the concept of the use of such devices only as a therapeutic intervention to treat a resident's medical condition, used after obtaining informed consent, and only if other less restrictive devices have been tried. Always rule out the possibility of an acute medical illness in residents whose presenting symptoms may be an increase in agitation or confusion or a change from their baseline behavioral state.

Remember that the restraint order must be based on the reason for applying the restraint, not just the type of restraint being used. All restraints in use must have an accompanying physician's order specifying the type, reason for use, release period, and exact time frame or situation use. Orders should not be vague or written as

TABLE 5.1   Concerns on the Use of Physical Restraints in Long-Term Care Facilities

- Is proper assessment of need documented?
- Have less restrictive techniques been tried prior to the ordering of a restraint?
- Is there a physician's order for the exact type and time frame for the restraint being used?
- Has the staff been properly trained in the use and monitoring of all restraint devices within the facility?
- Does the staff periodically release restraints on residents per policy guidelines and document the release schedule?
- Are restraints ordered that violate a resident's rights (no informed consent obtained)?
- Are restraints being ordered to prevent wandering or elopement?
- Is the correct size and type of restraint ordered for the resident?
- Is the continued need for restraints regularly reviewed?

TABLE 5.2   FDA Recommendations for Avoiding Hazards With Restraint Devices

- Assess why restraints are being considered and develop alternatives to restraint use; implement these alternatives before applying restraints.
- Use restraints *only* under the supervision of a licensed health care provider and for a strictly defined period of time.
- Define and communicate a clear institutional policy on the use of restraints. Include alternatives to restraints, appropriate conditions for use, and the length of time a restraint may be used in the policy. Make the policy available to residents and family members.
- Obtain informed consent from the resident or guardian before the use of restraints, unless an emergency situation exists.
- Display instructions for use of restraints in a visible location. Interpret in foreign languages as needed.
- Provide periodic in-service training for staff.
- Read and follow the manufacturer's directions before using restraints:
  - -select the appropriate type of restraint
  - -use the correct size
  - -note the "front" and "back" and apply restraints correctly
  - -secure restraints designed for use in bed to the springs or frame, *never* to the mattress or bed rails; if the bed is adjustable, secure restraints to parts of the bed that would move with the restrained individual
  - -tie knots with appropriate hitches so that they may be released quickly
- Emphasize good nursing, rehabilitative, and resident care practices:
  - -observe restrained individuals frequently
  - -remove restraints at least every two hours and more often if needed
  - -apply and adjust restraints properly to maintain body alignment and ensure resident comfort
  - -continue to assess restrained individuals; discontinue their use as soon as possible; consider restraints as a temporary solution only
- Clearly document the medical reason for the use of restraints, the type selected, and the length of time for treatment in the resident's chart.
- Follow all laws in your jurisdiction regarding the use of restraints.

Source: U.S. Food and Drug Administration (FDA). FDA safety alert: Potential hazards with restraint devices. Rockville, MD: Department of Health and Human Services, July 1992.

"restraint use prn resident safety" as the sole reason for their use. The Safe Medical Devices Act of 1990 requires all health care facilities to report to the Food and Drug Administration (FDA) and/or the manufacturer any adverse event in which a medical device, including restraints, may have caused or contributed to a resident's death or serious injury. This report must be made by the facility within 10 business days of becoming aware of the event.[7] The FDA recommendations for avoiding potential hazards with restraint devices are shown in Table 5.2.

All staff members and attending physicians need to be educated about the current federal and state guidelines for the use of restraints. Instruction regarding the facility's policy and alternatives to restraint use needs to be part of an ongoing process, and this training must be given to all new employees. Documentation of such training should be maintained in each employee's employment record.

NEUROPSYCHOACTIVE MEDICATIONS

The use of any centrally acting major or minor tranquilizer can cause potential side effects in an older, frail population. Table 5.3 lists medications with high risk for the older person. Although the use of antipsychotic medications (e.g., Haldol, Mellaril, Thorazine, and Navane) has been well established for the treatment of psychosis, the prescribing of these drugs for use with nonpsychotic behavioral disorders associated with dementia (agitation, wandering, repeated questioning, noisiness, hitting, and aggressive sexual behavior) has not.[8,9] However, it is common to see residents exhibiting these types of behavior as partial justification for the ordering of antipsychotic medications. The acceptable indications, per the

TABLE 5.3 Medications With High Risk for Central Nervous System Side Effects in the Older Person

Drug	*Effect*
• Analgesics	narcotics, indomethacin (Indocin), propoxyphene (Darvon)
• Antiemetics	trimethobenzamide (Tigan)
• Antihistamines	all medications with anticholinergic properties (e.g., diphenhydramine [Benadryl])
• Antipsychotics	all classes
• Antispasmodics	oxybutynin (Ditropan)
• Muscle relaxants	methocarbamol (Robaxin), carisoprodol (Soma)
• Sedative-hypnotics	all benzodiazepines

Omnibus Reconciliation Act (OBRA) guidelines, for the use of antipsychotics include:

- schizophrenia
- schizo-affective disorder
- delusional disorder
- psychotic mood disorder
- acute psychotic episodes
- brief reactive psychosis
- schizophreniform disorder
- atypical psychosis
- Tourette's syndrome
- Huntington's disease
- short-term (7 days) symptomatic treatment for hiccups, nausea, vomiting, or pruritus
- organic mental syndromes (including dementia and delirium) with associated psychotic and/or agitated behaviors that:
  (a) have been quantitatively and objectively documented
  (b) are not caused by preventable reasons
  (c) are causing the resident to present a danger to himself or herself or to others or result in a continuous cry, scream, yell, or pace, if these specific behaviors cause an impairment in functional capacity
  (d) are causing the resident to experience psychotic symptoms (hallucinations, paranoia, delusions) not exhibited as dangerous behaviors or as crying, screaming, yelling, or pacing, but which cause the resident distress or impairment in functional capacity

Antipsychotics should *not* be used if one or more of the following are the only indications for treatment: wandering, poor self-care, restlessness, impaired memory, anxiety, depression (without psychotic features), insomnia, unsociability, indifference to surroundings, fidgeting, nervousness, uncooperativeness, or agitated behaviors that do not represent danger to the resident or to others.

OBRA guidelines state:

The resident has the right to be free from any physical or chemical restraint imposed for purposes of discipline or convenience, and not required to treat the resident's medical symptoms.

Each resident's drug regimen must be free from unnecessary drugs which is defined by excessive dose, excessive duration, duplicate therapy, inadequate indications for its use or the presence of adverse consequences which indicate the dose should be reduced or discontinued.

The federal OBRA guidelines also require that an LTC facility:

- Document the specific condition or target symptoms, including psychiatric diagnoses, that warrant antipsychotic or other neuropsychoactive medication use
- Prohibit the use of antipsychotic medications if certain behaviors are the only justification (wandering, insomnia, or unsociability are not valid behavioral indications)
- Limit the use of antipsychotics on a "prn" basis (must have standing order for the same medication and use "prn" doses to control break-through symptoms)
- Monitor and document any untoward effects (e.g., decreased functional and mental status, movement disorders)
- Documentation of gradual dosage reductions coupled with attempts at behavioral programming. If unable to reduce dosage, document the reason why the reduction is not feasible or in the resident's best interest on a regular basis (at least every 6 months)

Appropriate consent must be obtained before any antipsychotic medication can be used. Such consent needs to be obtained regardless of the medical reason the medication is being prescribed so the resident or legal guardian can fully understand the risks and benefits of the administration of this class of drugs.

When short-acting benzodiazepines (short-acting forms are preferred in the older population) are prescribed for indications other than sleep induction, the following limitations should be considered:

1. Evidence exists that other possible reasons for the resident's distress have been considered and ruled out (including acute medical illness).
2. Such use results in a maintenance of or an improvement in the resident's functional status.
3. Daily use (at any dose) is less than 4 continuous months unless an attempt to a gradual dose reduction is unsuccessful.
4. Such use is for:
   - generalized anxiety disorders
   - organic mental syndromes (including dementia) with associated agitated states and which constitute a source of distress or dysfunction to the resident or represent a danger to the resident or others
   - panic disorders
   - symptomatic anxiety that occurs in residents with another diagnosed psychiatric disorder (e.g., depression, adjustment disorder) and use is equal to or less than the listed total daily doses allowed (see Table 5.4) (unless higher doses are medically necessary for the improvement or maintenance of the resident's functional status)

TABLE 5.4 Usual Total Daily Dosage for Short-Acting and Other
Anxiolytic Agents

Brand Name	Generic	Total Daily Oral Dosage for Older Persons
Ativan	lorazepam	2 mg
Serax	oxazepam	30 mg
Xanax	alprazolam	0.75 mg
Paxipam	halazepam	40 mg
BuSpar	buspirone HCL	30 mg
Atarax/Vistaril	hydroxyzine	50 mg
Many brands	chloral hydrate	750 mg

Both long- and short-acting benzodiazepines are limited to daily use of less than
4 continuous months unless an attempt at gradual dosage reduction is unsuccessful.
Beginning at 4 months, all residents should have dosage reductions considered for
this class of medication.

Risk management questions that must be addressed for any resident receiving
any neuropsychoactive medication include:

1. Has informed consent been obtained from the resident or guardian for
   antipsychotic or other neuropsychoactive medication use?
2. Is the behavior or condition significant enough to warrant medication?
3. Are there alternative interventions to the use of neuropsychoactive medications and have they been attempted?
4. Would a psychiatric evaluation be useful prior to initiation of therapy?
5. Is the medication appropriately prescribed for the condition and in the correct dosage? Are there any potential drug interactions for which the resident
   needs to be specifically monitored?
6. Is adequate blood monitoring (where applicable) ordered for the medication?
7. Is the staff monitoring for side effects and documenting the effect of the medication on the target symptoms?
8. Have specific goals of treatment been established?

The use of powerful neuropsychoactive medications in an LTC population
needs to be carefully monitored as the potential for serious side effects is significant. In-service education for licensed staff on the different classes of drugs and

their associated risks and benefits should be routinely offered for personnel of all shifts. Care plans should address the target behaviors for which therapy is being initiated, and the continued need for such medications should be routinely reevaluated and documented.

REFERENCES

1. Rubin BS, Dube AH, Mitchel EK. Asphysial deaths due to physical restraints. *Arch Fam Med.* 1993; 2:405–408.
2. Food and Drug Administration (FDA). FDA safety alert: Potential hazards with restraint devices. Rockville, MD: Department of Health and Human Services. July 1992.
3. Johnson SH. The fear of liability and the use of restraints in nursing homes. *Law, Medicine and Health Care.* 1990; 18(3):263–273.
4. Kapp MB. Nursing home restraints and legal liability. Merging the standard of care and industry practice. *J Legal Medicine.* 1992; 13:1–32.
5. Sloane PD, Papougenis D, Blakeslee J. Alternatives to physical and pharmacologic restraints in long-term care. *Am Family Physician.* 1992; 45:763–769.
6. Foltz-Gray D. Breaking free from restraints. *Contemp Longterm Care.* 1995; Jul:48–55.
7. The Safe Medical Devices Act of 1990, Pub. L. No. 101-629, 104 Stat. 4511 (1990). The user reporting provisions are contained in section 2(a).
8. Beers MD, Avorn J, Soumerai SB, et al. Psychoactive medication use in intermediate-care facility residents. *JAMA.* 1988; 260:3016–3020.
9. Smith DA. New rules for prescribing psychotropics in nursing homes. *Geriatrics.* 1990; 45:44–56.

10 Tips From This Chapter

1. Restraints should only be considered when less restrictive alternatives have been considered, tried, and failed. Always obtain informed consent.
2. Monitor all restraint interventions and audit documentation of their use on a regular basis.
3. Clearly document the medical reason for the use of restraints, the type selected, and the length of time for which they are to be used.
4. Electronic wristbands or other devices that trigger alarms are not considered restraints, but a resident has the right, if competent, to refuse to wear them.
5. A physician's order must always be obtained for the use of any restraint.
6. The resident has the right to be free from any physical or chemical restraint imposed for purposes of discipline or convenience and not required to treat the resident's medical symptoms.
7. Both long- and short-acting benzodiazepines are limited to daily use of less than 4 continuous months unless an attempt at gradual dosage reduction is unsuccessful.
8. Appropriate consent is needed before any antipsychotic medications can be used.
9. Ensure that all neuropsychoactive medications prescribed are appropriate for the condition and in the correct dosage. Always monitor for any potential drug interactions.
10. Ensure that staff monitor residents with prescribed neuropsychoactive medications for side effects and document the effect of the medication on the target symptoms.

6

Infection Control Issues

Infection control has always been a major concern for long-term care facilities. With the increasing number of admissions to the nursing home with infections of methicillin-resident *Staphylococcal aureus* (MRSA), *Clostridium difficile (C. difficile)*, vancomycin-resident *Enterococcus faecalis* (VREF), and other bacterial colonizers, the need to effectively address potential risk management issues for residents and staff alike has gained in importance in recent years.

All potential admissions should have their recent medical history reviewed for the presence of any of these organisms or other infectious agents, including tuberculosis (TB). If there appears to be any question of an active infection present, contact the referring facility and physician to obtain required information.

TB

Cases of TB have increased in the United States over the past decade, primarily due to the increase in HIV-related disease. However, reactivation of old TB pulmonary foci still accounts for most of the cases seen in the LTC setting. Routine annual screening (or more frequently, if clinically indicated) should be required of all staff and residents, with the results well documented. The Centers for Disease Control (CDC) issued its latest guidelines for preventing the spread of TB in health care settings in October 1994.[1] The CDC guidelines contained three major changes.

Risk Assessment

If facilities admit few, if any, residents with known TB, two new risk categories may now apply: "very low risk" and "minimal risk." These facilities need not have isolation rooms or other various ventilation systems present in the building. However, facilities falling into one of these two new categories must still

1. Have protocols for performing a risk assessment and identifying residents with suspected or known TB

2. Develop and periodically review a written TB infection control plan
3. Educate and counsel all health care workers in the facility
4. Conduct problem evaluation when TB transmission occurs
5. Report active TB cases to the public health department

Engineering

If isolation rooms are required for the facility, they must have at least 6 air changes per hour (ACH) and 12 ACH whenever feasible.

Respirators

The CDC recommends the use of National Institute of Occupational Safety and Health certified respirators (filtering masks) for health care workers exposed to infectious TB residents. However, the new high-efficiency particulate air respirators can meet this requirement as of August 1996, when the first 13 respirators were certified. These respirators will meet Occupational Safety and Health Administration (OSHA) requirements to protect health care workers from TB, although these devices must be fit-tested to obtain a face-seal leakage of 10% or less.

Each LTC facility should have a written TB infection control policy, including a respiratory protection program if clinically warranted, and all staff must be in-serviced on the content. Additional in-service programs should be held on TB, including the epidemiology, occupational risk, and work practices that may lessen exposure. The medical director may be an excellent resource to assist the infection control nurse in his or her role of monitoring for the presence of residents or staff with TB. All new admissions should be screened for the presence of possible TB infection using the two-step PPD test. If the results are equivocal, isolation of the resident is indicated until a complete evaluation can be done. For residents with known or suspected TB, all staff members entering the room or transporting a resident should wear OSHA-approved masks.

Preemployment PPD (or equivalent) skin testing and subsequent monitoring based on a risk assessment should be carried out on all potential employees. Any current employee who skin-converts from negative to positive should be thoroughly evaluated for active disease before being allowed to return to work. The arrangement for this evaluation and payment (if needed) are usually coordinated by the facility to ensure compliance. For all such converters, the infection control nurse should consider the possibility of nosocomial transmission and screen assigned residents of this employee to rule out active TB. It is critical that the facility's infection control nurse be familiar with all local and state health department TB guidelines and interface with public officials as required by law.

OTHER INFECTIOUS DISEASES

For residents with known or suspected MRSA, *C. difficile,* and VREF infections, proper surveillance cultures should be ordered as clinically indicated. Attempts should be made to cohort residents with similar bacterial colonizations whenever practicable in order to avoid infecting other residents with the organism. A written policy on the requirements for surveillance cultures should be developed with the input of the medical director and carried out under the supervision of the infection control nurse.

In-servicing all staff on the techniques and importance of good hand washing and other universal precautions should be completed on a regular basis. Classes also need to be made available for newly hired personnel, and documentation of such training is important. The key features of universal precautions are shown in Table 6.1.

The infection control nurse should report regularly to the medical board on the overall status of infections within the facility. This individual should also be responsible for the development and regular review of all facility policies for the safe handling of potentially infectious body fluids or contaminated linen and clothing. These policies should also be in-serviced to all staff members. For facilities accepting HIV residents, universal precautions should cover the main infection control requirements, although specific policies may need to be developed for each facility.

VACCINE PROGRAMS

The administration and documentation of pneumonia and influenza vaccines for residents need to be systematically organized and implemented. A complete vaccination history should be obtained for all new admissions. In general, pneumonia vaccines can be safely given to residents where the past administration is unknown or unclear. Both pneumonia and influenza vaccines have been shown to decrease morbidity and mortality in an older, frail population. Other vaccinations, such as tetanus, should also be kept current, and a written policy should be developed, with the input of the medical director, concerning all recommended vaccines.

FOOD-RELATED ISSUES

Food preparation and storage are a critical aspect of infection control and are often cited by inspectors on surveys as an area of deficiency in many LTC facilities. Many bacterial strains, such as *Salmonella* and *E. coli,* can be a common cause of food-borne illness in a nursing home. Most food-related illnesses are due to

TABLE 6.1   Key Features of Universal Precautions

- Wear gloves (change after each resident encounter) when coming into contact with any body secretions or contaminated items.
- Wear gowns/masks and eye protection as clinically indicated.
- Good hand washing techniques are required after each resident encounter.
- Label rooms appropriately to inform visitors to seek staff assistance before entering (respect confidentiality).
- Dispose of all body fluids and contaminated linens or clothing in accordance with current CDC guidelines.
- Label and package appropriately all containers that have potentially infectious material inside and ensure that proper disposal is carried out.

residents ingesting contaminated and undercooked beef, egg, and poultry products. All meats and poultry should be thoroughly cooked before serving and kept at an appropriate temperature during transportation to the units. For any suspected outbreak of food-borne illness within a facility, contact the local health department early to assist the facility in tracking the epidemiology of the outbreak.

Kitchens and refrigerators should be routinely inspected by facility supervisors to ensure personnel are properly preparing and storing food products. Foods should not be left uncovered in preparation areas or in refrigerators, and storage in residents' rooms should not be allowed unless food items are stable at room temperature and are properly sealed. Also, food should not be left at the nurses' station. The temperature settings of all freezers and refrigerators should be routinely checked with a thermometer.

ACUTE ILLNESS/EPIDEMICS

The attending physician should be notified if any resident exhibits even a subtle change in his or her baseline condition. Low-grade temperature elevations may represent early, serious infections and can also lead to dehydration.[2,3] If a resident with a known infectious process does not appear to be responding to the current treatment, the attending physician should be requested to reevaluate the prescribed therapy. Treatment of fevers with acetaminophen may only serve to obscure the clinical course of an impending infection.[4] Outside referral to the acute care hospital emergency department should be seriously considered for all residents appearing to be septic.

For possible epidemics of infectious disease within a facility, notify the medical director as soon as possible so that he or she can assist in the overall coordination of the evaluation and treatment of the outbreak. The medical director is the backup physician when the primary attending physician of record cannot be reached or is not responding appropriately to the decline in a resident's condition. All outbreaks of diarrheal disease or other flulike syndromes should be thoroughly and promptly investigated for the possibility of a facilitywide epidemic. Lawsuits against facilities in which residents have died from epidemic illness have named the medical director as a codefendant based on his or her alleged lack of supervision of the facility's and physician's response to the infectious outbreak.

Infectious disease needs to be addressed in an organized manner, and acute illnesses should be promptly investigated and appropriately treated. For residents with serious illness not responding to initial prescribed therapy, referral to an acute care setting may be necessary in order to reduce morbidity and mortality. Education of all staff on the many aspects of infection control is highly recommended and can help the facility maintain an effective approach to infection control issues.

REFERENCES

1. Centers for Disease Control and Prevention. *Fed Regist.* 1994 Oct 28; 59(208):54242–54303.
2. Pals JK, Weinberg AD, Beal LF, et al. Clinical Triggers for Detection of Fever and Dehydration: Implications for Long-Term Care Nursing. *Gerontol Nurs.* 1995; 21:13–19.
3. Castle SC, Norman DC, Yeh M, et al. Fever response in elderly nursing home-residents: Are the older truly colder? *J Am Geriatr Soc.* 1991; 39:853–857.
4. Weinberg AD, Pals JK, McGlinchey-Berroth R. The source of fever and the effect of acetaminophen use on time to diagnosis in febrile long-term care residents. *Nurs Home Med.* 1996; 4:340–347.

10 Tips From This Chapter

1. Annual TB monitoring of all residents and staff should be performed and documented.
2. The facility's written TB policy should be in-serviced to all staff. Certified protective respiratory masks should be available for use by staff when caring for all residents with known or suspected TB.
3. Screen all potential admissions for the presence of TB, *C. difficile,* VREF and MRSA infections. If in doubt, call the referring facility.
4. Stress that proper universal precautions must be utilized by staff with all residents and emphasize good hand washing techniques.
5. Always contact the attending physician for all fevers lasting more than 24 hours, even if low grade, as they may represent early serious infection and can cause dehydration if untreated.
6. Regularly inspect the kitchen for cleanliness and for proper preparation, storage, and refrigeration of all foods.
7. The medical director should be involved any time there is a suspected or known infectious epidemic within the facility.
8. Pneumonia and influenza vaccine programs should be encouraged for all appropriate residents and documented accurately.
9. The facility's infection control nurse should routinely report to the medical board on the current status of any infections in the facility and work with designated personnel to develop interventions for all potential risk management issues.
10. The medical director should be contacted any time a resident appears not to be responding to a prescribed intervention for an infection or the attending physician is not available or is unresponsive to nursing inquiries.

7

Prevention of Resident Neglect or Abuse

Even with the myriad of federal and state regulations concerning resident rights that are in force nowadays, abuse can still occur in the nursing home setting. Since 1975, when the Older Americans Act was passed, the state Ombudsman programs were established to respond to the issue of neglect and abuse of long-term care residents. Subsequently, health care providers in all 50 states are required by law to report each and every instance of suspected abuse. Nursing home residents seem particularly vulnerable to abuse, and Table 7.1 lists the major reasons this occurs. The most common scenario is the permanent assignment of one staff member on a shift to a cognitively impaired individual (i.e., an individual exhibiting any dementing illness) who verbally or physically abuses staff from time to time. Exact statistics on the prevalence of staff abuse of residents is not yet available, but it is probably more prevalent than generally believed. The majority of alleged incidents appear to occur on night shifts when the number of supervisory personnel may be limited.

Residents of nursing homes have rights protected by state and federal statutes. These include the right to

- participate in all health care decisions
- give informed consent for all treatments and medications
- refuse all pharmacological and physical restraints
- have access to a long-term care ombudsman or equivalent representative
- have access to a personal physician 365 days a year
- be free of all verbal, mental, physical, or sexual abuse
- be free of all corporal punishment
- be free from involuntary seclusion unless specifically ordered by an attending physician for documented reasons

TABLE 7.1   Major Indicators of Potential Resident Abuse in the Nursing Home Setting

1. Infrequent or no visitation by family members
2. Very low staff-to-resident ratios leading to increased fatigue and stress on the part of the caregiver
3. Abusive residents with high care needs assigned to the same staff person
4. Inadequately trained and supervised nursing home staff, especially on evening and night shifts
5. High rates of staff turnover each year
6. Facilities with poor working conditions and/or low salary or benefit levels
7. Obvious burnout among staff members

Every facility must make a concerted effort to detect and prevent nursing home resident neglect and abuse. It is important that the staff understand that residents with dementia who become aggressive are not intentional in their behavior. Furthermore, this behavior never justifies retaliation by an employee toward the resident. Many lawsuits against LTC facilities specifically mention neglect and abuse in the actual complaint and use the medical record to justify any such accusation. The directors of nursing and medical director can help monitor the facility for any possible neglect or abuse by seeking answers to some basic identification questions:

1. On rounds in the facility, do residents appear to have unexplained bruises over their bodies?
2. Have families reported incidents where their relatives claim they were hit or otherwise abused during any shift, particularly nights?
3. Is there any evidence to suggest that staff members yell or swear at residents?
4. Do some residents appear agitated or try to avoid contact with a particular staff member?
5. Do some staff members appear to have a persistent angry attitude or manner?
6. Are residents wearing restraints that appear to have been placed too tightly for longer than authorized time periods?

Although you can make every possible effort, there may occasionally be personnel who will be responsible for abuse of residents. These incidents must be thoroughly and completely investigated and any identified abusers among staff must be terminated immediately. It is, of course, prudent to transfer any alleged abuser to another ward when possible to allow for a more open investigation and to prevent retribution against the victim during the investigative process. It is important that your facility have a policy concerning the investigation of any alleged complaints of abuse and that all staff members have been required to review and sign the policy before being allowed to work in the facility.

Table 7.2 lists the recommended methods of documenting alleged abuse of a nursing home resident. Appropriate notification, documentation, investigation, and follow-up is critical if the truth is to be discovered and future incidents prevented. A full history and physical exam should be performed by the attending physician (or appropriate designee) as soon as possible, and all ordered laboratory tests and x-rays should be recorded. It is helpful if a specific form is developed by a facility for this purpose. The basic elements that such a form should incorporate are shown in Figure 7.1.

Although exact statistics are not available, sexual abuse exists in the nursing home setting. The possibility of sexual abuse should be investigated during all suspected abuse cases and, when confirmed, should be promptly reported to all legally required agencies. Sexual abuse of a nursing home resident may be associated with the following signs and symptoms:

- Extreme fear of a particular staff member
- Fear of getting undressed
- Difficulty in sitting or walking
- Irritation of the genital or rectal areas not explained on the basis of medical illness
- Torn, bloody, or stained underwear
- Ripped bed garments that are not readily explainable
- Unexplained genital infections

Family members should be encouraged to come forward with questions regarding the care of their relatives and attempt to obtain answers for unexplained bruises or other injuries. If they are unhappy with the explanation being given by the staff, family members should be urged to speak to the director of nursing or the nursing home administrator. In no way should inquiries be dismissed out of hand without investigation.

In recent judgments neglect has been interpreted by juries to cover a large number of difficult problems affecting nursing home residents, including failure to monitor weight with resulting weight loss, failure to continue physical therapy even though maximal recovery appears to have been attained, failure to turn a resident every 2 hours as ordered, failure to provide adequate treatment for a pressure ulcer, and inadequate staffing to provide required services on all shifts 7 days a week.

Table 7.3 lists intervention strategies that can be employed by a facility's administrative staff to keep abreast of potential abuse and ways to deal with the problem in the nursing home setting.

An ongoing challenge is to minimize or prevent burnout and allow staff members to appropriately vent their frustrations. It is critical that charge nurses or super-

(continued on p. 42)

TABLE 7.2   Documentation of Alleged Abuse of a Long-Term Care
Resident

1. Notify the facility's director of nursing, nursing home administrator, and medical director immediately.
2. Notify all state and local officials as required by regulation/law.
3. Completely document the alleged incident in the resident's own words with details regarding time and alleged personnel involved.
4. Have the attending physician or other assigned health care practitioner perform a physical exam (including a mental status examination) as soon as possible in order to document the presence of any injuries that could substantiate a claim. This exam must be done immediately and not postponed until the time of the next regularly scheduled visit by the attending physician.
5. Document the results of all ordered laboratory tests and x-rays subsequent to the injuries being noted.
6. During the physical exam:
   - undress the resident, using modesty drapes, to assess for any potential injuries
   - record all bruises, lacerations, and contusions as to size, type, location, number, and stage of healing
   - check for sexual abuse
7. Obtain photographs (preferably in color) to document all physical exam findings. First, obtain permission from the resident (if competent) or legal guardian (if resident is incompetent to give consent). These photographs should be taken with a minimum of two shots per injured area, from different angles, and prior to medical treatment of the injuries if possible. The date and time should be included on the pictures.
8. Compare injuries to staff progress notes to determine if there is a possible explanation for the injuries seen.
9. Document all interventions, medical treatments, and follow-up orders.
10. Record the names of officials (state or local) to whom anyone at the facility may have spoken.

Adapted from Weinberg AD, Wei J, (Eds.). *The Early Recognition of Elder Abuse: A Quick Reference Guide.* Copyright © 1995 American Medical Publishing Co., Inc., Bayside, NY. Reprinted by permission of the publisher.

I. History and Background Information

1. History of present illness for which resident was admitted to the nursing home:

_____

_____

2. Alleged abuse or neglect as stated by the resident:

_____

_____

3. Cognitive or physical impairments of resident:

_____

_____

4. Recent conflicts or incidents involving resident and staff:

_____

_____

5. Can the resident recall any instances of:
   - ( ) rough handling
   - ( ) slapping or hitting
   - ( ) yelling
   - ( ) threats
   - ( ) excessive restraint use
   - ( ) isolation/confinement
   - ( ) misuse/theft of property or money
   - ( ) staff refusal to help feed
   - ( ) staff refusal to help with hygiene needs
   - ( ) sexual abuse

6. Interview process:
   Review:
   - ( ) staff activities during the date and shift in question
   - ( ) presence of denial, blaming resident, or excessive defensiveness
   - ( ) staff members' recollection of alleged incident
   - ( ) witnessed accounts of any threatening or abusive acts
   - ( ) statements of relatives/friends

II. Physical Examination and Findings

BP _____ Weight _____ Pulse _____ Respiratory rate _____

1. General appearance (including personal hygiene)

_____

2. Current mental status exam and overall behavior during exam

_____

FIGURE 7.1 Nursing home resident abuse/neglect protocol.

3. Any evidence of physical neglect (dehydration, malnourishment, poor grooming)

———

4. Any evidence of physical abuse (including defensive injuries on extensor surfaces of arms)

———

( ) Head/eye injuries _____
( ) Friction/restraint injuries _____
( ) Laceration injuries _____
( ) Sprains/dislocations _____
( ) Unexplained bruises _____
      ( ) face, lips, mouth
      ( ) torso, back, buttocks
      ( ) upper arms
      ( ) clustered, forming patterns
      ( ) similar to a striking object (e.g., bed rail)
      ( ) multiple in various stages of healing
( ) Other injuries noted _____

5. Any evidence of psychological abuse

———

6. Any evidence of sexual abuse

———

III. Diagnostics
1. Color photos taken at _____ AM/PM.
   • Label with name, date, photographer, witness; include in picture a ruler by the lesions and picture of patient's face.
2. Laboratory data (as clinically indicated):
   • Complete blood count
   • Urinalysis, serum electrolytes, blood urea nitrogen, and creatinine (dehydration)
   • GC, VDRL, and chlamydia cultures (sexual abuse)
   • Radiological screening for fractures (physical abuse)
   • Metabolic screening for nutritional abnormalities (e.g., total protein, albumin)
   • CT scan of head (known or suspected head trauma or major change in neurological status)

FIGURE 7.1   (continued)

IV. Assessment

( ) No evidence for any form of abuse

( ) Evidence for psychological abuse (verbal, threats, isolation)

( ) Evidence of physical abuse (deliberate, inappropriate care, direct beating or slapping)

( ) Evidence for sexual abuse

( ) Evidence for physical neglect by staff

Medical findings are consistent with _____

Agency/authorities contacted (include date and time):

_____

Facility personnel notified:		FOLLOW-UP:
Medical director:	_____	_____
Director of nursing:	_____	_____
Administrator:	_____	_____
Family contacted:	_____	_____

Adapted from Weinberg AD, Wei J, (Eds.): *The Early Recognition of Elder Abuse: A Quick Reference Guide.* Copyright © 1995 American Medical Publishing Co., Inc., Bayside, NY. Reprinted by permission of the publisher.

FIGURE 7.1 (continued)

TABLE 7.3 Intervention Strategies in the Nursing Home Setting

1. Conduct anonymous surveys among staff to detect participation in resident abuse or neglect.
2. Instruct all staff members that resident abuse or neglect will not be tolerated and post formal written policies on how the facility will deal with reports of alleged neglect and/or abuse. In-service all staff on these policies.
3. Organize special training in conflict resolution or "venting" sessions where staff members can express frustration with their jobs or with working with difficult/abusive residents.
4. Rotate aides and nurses working with difficult or abusive residents on a regular basis.

TABLE 7.3   (continued)

5. Meet with any family members who have voiced complaints of poor care on the part of the staff toward their relative.

6. Hold regular in-service sessions for all shifts on how to better understand the abusive actions of nursing home residents toward staff and on how to depersonalize the conflict.

7. Hold regular in-service sessions for all shifts on dealing with cultural and ethnic differences of the resident population. Offer suggestions on developing coping mechanisms.

8. Immediately involve the resident's attending physician and the facility's medical director when alleged complaints of neglect or abuse are filed or suspected.

9. Involve the psychiatric liaison nurse or consultant psychiatrist in helping the staff to manage:
   - difficult or aggressive residents
   - residents who appear to have suffered abuse or neglect
   - incident debriefing sessions for members of staff following a reported case of neglect/abuse

10. Attempt to improve the general morale of the staff (e.g., special recognition day, remembering them at holiday times, thank-you notes for any job well done, include staff in policy/decision making to involve them in the institution).

Adapted from Weinberg AD, Wei J, (Eds.): *The Early Recognition of Elder Abuse: A Quick Reference Guide.* Copyright © 1995 American Medical Publishing Co., Inc., Bayside, NY. Reprinted by permission of the publisher.

visors immediately report any signs of attitude or emotional distress concerning staff so that care assignments can be reevaluated or rotated. The use of stress-reduction groups and other in-service programs on understanding and dealing with abusive residents can also be extremely helpful. It is important that such programs be available to staff members of all shifts and that these programs be repeated on a regular basis.

Some facilities have used psychiatric liaison nurses or the consulting psychiatrist in helping the staff to manage not only difficult or aggressive residents but also the staff's reaction to caring for them. Such consultants may prove invaluable if an actual incident occurs as they may conduct an incident debriefing session for all staff. Many facilities have tried to improve and/or maintain the general morale of the staff at a high level by fostering special recognition days, remembering staff at holiday time, sending personalized thank-you notes for any job well done, and making a special effort to include staff in all major policy and decision-making activities.

To summarize, almost all resident abuse by staff is preventable. However, it involves a dedicated administrator and an ongoing facilitywide program to affirm staff awareness of this potential problem and to address any staff tensions/issues that may be a symptom of possible impending conflicts. Constant vigilance is required on the part of all staff to report any possible abuse or neglect to the supervisor so that action may be initiated immediately.

---

10 Tips From This Chapter

1. Assume all alleged abuse is true until proven otherwise.
2. Avoid assigning the same staff member to an abusive/agitated resident on a regular basis. Rotate difficult assignments.
3. Officially notify the designated state office and the facility's medical director of all alleged incidents. Involve local police as each situation warrants.
4. Have supervisory personnel make unannounced rounds on nights and weekends.
5. Provide recurrent in-service offerings on dealing with the agitated and/or abusive resident and similar staff "venting" sessions.
6. Document all investigations conducted when a complaint is made.
7. Residents who have a high acuity of care needs and for whom proper staffing to supply those needs is not always possible should be considered for transfer to another facility.
8. Stress in staff meetings that no form of verbal, physical, or psychological abuse will be tolerated and that such abuse will be cause for immediate dismissal without a letter of recommendation.
9. Stress the importance of documentation for all unexplained injuries of residents.
10. Keep families informed of all relevant findings. A wall of silence will only make relatives more suspicious and will usually cause them to seek outside help.

8

Falls and Resident Safety Concerns

Accidents remain the fifth leading cause of death for persons over 65, and approximately two-thirds of these are directly related to falls and their consequences. The frail older adult is at higher risk for falling than other people of similar age and is also prone to other types of injuries. This chapter will review some of the more important aspects of resident safety.

WANDERING AND ELOPEMENT

Among the many concerns regarding safety issues in the long-term care environment, wandering and elopement remain potentially the most dangerous situation a facility can face.[1,2,3] Elopements, which involve purposeful and repeated attempts of a resident to leave the facility, are often more difficult to control than random wandering into stairwells or other potentially unsafe areas.

Because physical restraint use has declined and because the use of locked doorways and exits is strictly limited by local and state fire codes, wandering and elopement should be addressed by behavioral and other modifications to the physical structure of the unit and building whenever possible. Approximately 70% of elopement claims involve a resident death that occurred as a result of the event, and such lawsuits represent about 10% of all legal actions initiated against LTC facilities.[4]

The vast majority of elopements involve residents already identified as elopement risks. Often this determination can be made by the staff within a few days of admission. Thus, care plans and other preventive measures can be utilized to decrease or prevent injuries to these residents due to elopement-related incidents. Care plans must be revised as often as required by clinical changes in each resident's condition.

Identification of a resident at risk for wandering and elopement can begin during the admission process by reviewing any medical records sent with the resident from previous health care providers and by interviewing (via telephone or in person) appropriate family members. Standard questions should include the following:

- Is wandering a current problem?
- Are there certain time periods during the day in which wandering behavior is more prevalent?
- Are there possible physical reasons why wandering occurs (e.g., related to hunger, pain, or need to urinate)?
- What effective interventions can best redirect the behavior?

Since almost half of all elopements occur within the first 48 hours following admission to an LTC facility, all staff members need to pay particular attention to the whereabouts of a new resident during this period and for the subsequent week at least. Wandering behaviors can best be classified into several areas[5]:

1. Escapist wanderer (eloper)
2. Purposeful wanderer
3. Aimless wanderer
4. Critical wanderer (cannot differentiate safe from unsafe situations)

To balance the rights of the resident while providing the least restrictive yet protective living environment, certain risk prevention strategies need to be employed. Because controlled wandering can assist residents in achieving some form of exercise and relief of tension, suppression of wandering activity should never be the primary goal of any such program. Recommendations to manage wandering include the following:

- Maintain adequate lighting in all corridors.
- Provide a scheduled exercise or walking program to reduce nocturnal wandering.
- Design meaningful group activities to keep the residents involved in interesting projects.
- Designate a secure walking area where residents can ambulate in safety.
- Place arrows on the floor that lead in a complete circle to allow the residents to follow them as part of a walking program.
- Keep clocks and calendars (large type) in common areas to assist in the residents' orientation to time and date.
- Encourage family and friends to visit the residents.
- Use videotapes of family members to calm the residents during periods of agitated wandering.
- Provide as much continuity of care as possible by assigning staff to the care of the same residents.

- Have staff use one-to-one redirection for confused and wandering residents.
- Electronic alarm systems can be helpful adjuncts in any preventive program, but staff must be fully trained in their proper use and limitations.
- Have the pharmacy consultant review all medication profiles of wandering residents to ensure that no medication may be precipitating or exaggerating any existing symptomatology.
- Use snacks to help redirect wandering residents.
- Hold regular in-service programs to increase staff awareness of the risks for wandering residents.
- For any identified residents with known wandering tendencies, have care plans carefully address this issue and then follow those plans (modify as needed).
- Residents prone to wandering should have their rooms located, if possible, near the nursing station.
- Establish facilitywide protocols that will effectively aid staff in conducting checks on wandering-prone residents.
- Minimize the use of physical restraints.
- Develop and regularly in-service all staff on a facilitywide plan regarding the management of wandering residents and the search for missing residents.

All facilities should develop and test a formal protocol to find residents who are missing from their units. Also, all staff members should be prepared to mobilize to locate a missing resident, not just the personnel from the ward where the resident lives.[6] A sample protocol is shown in Table 8.1.

Liability issues that need to be addressed in an LTC facility regarding the dangers of wandering and elopement include the following[7]:

- Does the facility have adequate safeguards in place to prevent a resident from eloping without detection by staff?
- Does the facility identify those residents at risk for elopement? Has this been noted on their care plans?
- Does the facility have policies and procedures in place to prevent elopements from occurring? Are staff members able to implement them correctly when needed?
- Does the facility maintain adequate staffing to safeguard those with a tendency to wander or elope?

RESIDENT ASSAULTS AGAINST OTHER RESIDENTS

Resident-to-resident assaults do occur and can result in legal claims against the facility. The assaults often involve residents with dementia or cognitive impairment from neurovascular diseases, which culminate in arguments with other resi-

TABLE 8.1 Protocol to Locate a Missing Resident

If a resident is thought to be missing, begin by investigating alternative explanations (e.g., on a pass, at a medical appointment, on a field trip, or at a facility activity). If the resident's absence cannot be explained, assume that he or she is missing. Then:

1. Notify all staff that a resident is missing. Determine the last time the resident was seen and what clothing he or she was wearing. Determine the last area of the building in which the resident was seen and search that area carefully.
2. Call for additional staff as needed to help locate the resident. A search coordinator should be responsible for all aspects of the search.
3. Notify management (the director of nursing, the administrator, and others as required by facility policy).
4. Extend the search to cover the entire facility, including other residents' rooms and the entire grounds of the facility. Investigate all departments, closets, mechanical areas, bathrooms, offices, and other areas usually kept locked.
5. Notify the local police or fire department and request their assistance if the resident may have wandered off the grounds. Prepare a missing resident profile for their use.
6. Notify family members and request their assistance, if appropriate (they might have an idea where a resident may have wandered to).
7. Notify state agencies as required by regulations.
8. When the resident is found, examine him or her for any injuries and arrange treatment, if required.
9. Complete an incident report, if required, and document the entire incident.
10. Call the attending physician if the resident cannot be located or if injuries are suspected when he or she is found. Request orders to arrange for emergency evaluation if serious injury is suspected.

dents and can subsequently escalate to violence. The redirection of such escalating behavior and the separation of residents involved in arguments are necessary steps in controlling this situation. Additionally, screening applicants carefully for a history of violent behavior prior to their admission to the facility can help determine the facility's ability to offer safe and proper care for those residents and to provide for the safety of other residents.

For those residents identified as having a tendency to be violent, determining any initiating or escalating factors is important. The staff should be trained to avoid these factors whenever possible. Care plans also need to fully address these issues. Completing all required incident reports, involving the attending physician, officially notifying local police of assaults, and contacting appropriate family members should routinely be done in all assault cases.

If injuries are suspected as a result of an assault, seek appropriate evaluation and treatment immediately. If any particular resident appears to be unsafe to remain in the facility due to violent-prone behavior, transfer to a more appropriate facility must be considered by the interdisciplinary care team. The involvement of the psychiatric consultant can be extremely helpful in these often difficult situations.

FALLS

Falls remain an ongoing concern for all facilities. The older the individual, the greater the chance that a negative outcome will result from any fall. Also, a history of repeated falls is often a major factor in why someone is first admitted to an LTC facility. On average, a nursing home resident falls approximately twice a year.[8,9] These falls may be due to a variety of issues.[10] All residents with a history of falling or documented falls within the facility need to have their fall risk assessed and have the care plan address this issue. In fact, all residents should have a fall risk assessment completed at the time of admission to the facility. This assessment should be reviewed and updated at regular intervals.

Resident falls remain among the most frequent claims reported to insurance companies covering LTC facilities, and these claims are increasing in cost to the carriers. Appropriate nursing home policies dealing with falls and fall prevention should be available and the staff appropriately in-serviced on them.[11] Nursing home fall assessment instruments are available. The major categories to be assessed in these instruments are shown in Table 8.2.

Most falls occur at the bedside, often when a resident is transferring to or from the bed. Bed monitors that sound an alarm when a resident attempts to get out of bed are not wholly reliable and do not replace adequate supervision of the resident. Restraints have no role in preventing falls, as the majority of individuals being restrained actually end up falling at times when the restraint is removed.

The most frequent risk factors contributing to falls are:

- confusion
- unstable cardiovascular condition (with hypotension or orthostatic changes)
- decreased mobility in the lower extremities
- general weakness
- elimination needs
- orthopedic problems or a reliance on assistive devices
- visual problems
- severe arthritis or other joint problems

Age alone does not determine who will or will not fall. Residents of any age who believe they are fairly independent are less likely to ask for help may thus increase their risk of falling. Intervention plans to address fall risk must be inter-

TABLE 8.2   Major Categories to Be Addressed in a Falls
Assessment Instrument

- Mental status
- Length of stay
- Elimination (incontinence problems)
- History of falling
- Visual impairment
- Gait and balance
- Use of assistive devices for ambulation
- Use of wheelchairs and proper transferring technique
- History of orthostatic blood pressure changes
- Change in functional status
- Medications prescribed:

- sedatives	*- hypnotics*	*- anti-Parkinsonian drugs*
- antihistamines	*- sedatives/hypnotics*	*- benzodiazepines*
- psychotropics	*- antiseizure/antiepileptics*	*- narcotics*

disciplinary in nature and be reassessed as clinical needs dictate. Ways to reduce the risk of falling are shown in Table 8.3. It is imperative that maintenance personnel routinely monitor and correct any environmental safety hazards that could contribute to falls (e.g., areas under repair, loose flooring, leaking roofs, and broken handrails). Additionally, ongoing data collection to be used in the analysis of high-risk areas and times can be helpful in the revision of the current fall-prevention program to address any identified problem areas.

FIRE

Training all staff members on proper procedures in the eventuality of a fire must be considered a very high priority. Mock evacuations, if not mandated by local statute, should be done on a regular basis to heighten the awareness of the staff to possible complications of moving residents in an emergency situation. In-servicing of all newly hired staff on proper fire safety needs must also be done.

SMOKING ISSUES

Although many facilities have no-smoking policies, residents generally are still able to smoke at certain times in designated areas, often just outside a facility. However, the risk of injury to the resident or the starting of a fire in the building is always a potentially disastrous possibility.

TABLE 8.3 Strategies to Lower Fall Risk

- Identify residents at high risk for falling and address interventions in their care plan.
- Minimize restraint use and keep residents active and ambulating as much as possible.
- Encourage residents to ask for help when rising.
- Encourage residents to wear proper shoes and use canes and walkers as instructed.
- Encourage weight bearing when transferring a resident.
- Minimize any medications with sedative side effects and do not use sedatives as a fall-prevention strategy.
- For those with cardiovascular instability, encourage them to rise slowly from a sitting position.
- Maintain adequate hydration.
- Encourage the use of necessary prescription eyeglasses to decrease visual impairment.
- Clean up any wet areas immediately; use warning signs when cleaning floors.
- Provide adequate lighting in all rooms and common areas.
- Carpet all high-fall risk areas to help reduce severity of injuries from falls.
- Keep all areas free of debris and objects that may cause residents to fall.
- Install and properly maintain handrails in all resident areas.
- Provide assistance for all residents going to and from the bathroom.
- Ensure that all visitors of residents at risk for falling are aware of any nursing guidelines and care plan interventions.
- Install grab bars in all bathrooms and use elevated toilet seats when needed.

For those residents with impaired mental status who are allowed to smoke per the facility's policy, proper supervision of smoking materials, matches, and the actual smoking area is required. Also, because mental status can change over time, periodic reevaluation of the smoking safety of a resident may need to be done. For some residents, the use of a smoking tunic (made of flame-retardant fiberglass cloth) may be an added safety feature. Such tunics cost less than $25. Family members who visit need to be fully aware of the facility's smoking policy and must adhere to it. Additionally, all staff members need to be aware of the facility's rules and regulations and the degree of supervision required for each resident assigned to them on any particular day.

EMPLOYEE WORKPLACE RISK FACTORS

Employee injuries can occur from a variety of sources in a nursing home. The identification of high-risk areas and procedures (e.g., lifting bed-bound residents) needs to be incorporated into the routine orientation of new employees. The Occupational Safety and Health Administration has a myriad of rules to protect workers from environmental hazards. A staff member of the facility should be designated as the employee safety coordinator and should become familiar with all applicable standards and guidelines.

The medical director of the facility should be aware of all potential hazardous areas in the building during weekly rounds. He or she should then document that these areas are properly marked and inaccessible to residents. Physicals are sometimes performed by the medical director during the hiring process to screen for major illnesses, and employees with specific health concerns (e.g., previous back injuries or history of orthopedic surgery) can be offered counseling to lessen the risk of future injury on the job. Some nursing home facilities may alternatively require that a physical be completed by an applicant's private physician.

REFERENCES

1. Harwood G, McGlenister E. Wandering patients: Potential for tragedy. *Leadership.* 1993; 2(1):30–33.
2. Rodriguez J. Resident falls and elopements. Costs and controls. *Nurs Homes.* 1993; 42(4):16–17.
3. Top claim concerns: Falls, wandering, delayed treatment. In *Nursing Home Update.* St. Paul, MN: St. Paul Fire and Marine Insurance Co., 1994.
4. Rajecki R. Stake a claim for safety. Program highlights risk reduction. *Contemp Long Term Care.* 1991; 14(4):42–43, 72–73.
5. Butler JP, Barnett CA. Window of wandering. *Geriatr Nurs.* 1991; 12(5):226–227.
6. Rader J. A comprehensive staff approach to problem wandering. *Gerontologist.* 1987; 27(6):756–760.
7. Rozovsky LE, Rozovsky FA. Legal implications when residents elope. *Long Term Care.* 1986; March: 6–7.
8. Robbins AS, Rubenstein LZ, Josephson KR, et al. Predictors of falls among elderly people: Results of two population based studies. *Arch Intern Med.* 1989; 149:1628–1633.
9. Wells BG, Middleton B, Lawrence G, et al. Factors associated with the elderly falling in intermediate care facilities. *Drug Intell Clin Pharm.* 1985; 19:142–145.
10. Lipsitz LA. Clinical crossroads: An 85-year-old woman with a history of falls. *JAMA.* 1996; 276:59–66.
11. Strumf NE, Wagner J, Evans LK, et al. *Reducing Restraints: Individual Approaches to Behavior.* Huntington Valley, PA: The Whitman Group, 1992.

10 Tips From This Chapter

1. Identify all potential wanderers/elopement risks within 3 days of admission and add this issue to the care plan and problem list. Ensure this information is given to the personnel caring for this resident.
2. Establish protocols to deal with missing residents and use practice drills to educate the staff on their implementation. In-service all new employees on these protocols.
3. If electronic devices and alarms are used, ensure that adequate training is given to all personnel. Train new staff members on their use prior to allowing them on the floor. Instruct staff to *always* investigate each time such an alarm is triggered.
4. Ensure that all staff are in-serviced on proper documentation of missing residents and on the facility's policies on handling elopements.
5. Develop alternative behavioral and environmental modifications to allow wandering to continue in a controlled setting (check local fire and safety codes). Involve the recreational therapy department in these programs when possible.
6. Identification of potentially violent residents is a priority. Orientation, redirection, and separation of residents involved in arguments are the primary approaches to avoiding resident-to-resident assaults.
7. Early identification of residents at high risk for falling should be done after admission and addressed in the nursing care plan. Reevaluate the risk for falling on a regular basis as clinical conditions warrant.
8. Develop procedures for the assessment, reassessment, monitoring, and reporting of all resident falls, including a resident fall assessment tool.
9. Provide ongoing education to all residents, families, and staff on falls and fall-prevention strategies.
10. Smoking policies should be known to residents, visitors, and staff. Practice fire safety and disaster evacuation drills on a regular basis.

9

The Role of the Medical Director

The medical director of a facility can play a critical role in helping the staff to maintain a high level of quality care and to reduce legal exposure to potential acts of negligence and malpractice. Many facilities do not do an exhaustive search for their medical director and most often are satisfied just to find someone to fill the position. This approach can be foolish in the long run and should be avoided.

The medical director serves as the physician liaison with all other physicians and health care practitioners working in a facility. He or she can communicate problems as they arise and facilitate solutions. While it may be difficult to find a qualified, competent physician to serve as medical director, it is not impossible.

When a current medical director departs a facility, the usual way a replacement is chosen is to ask one of the other attending physicians if he or she would like to assume the role. Since the requirements of this position mandate that the medical director be available 24 hours a day, 365 days a year for emergencies, the usual pay range of $250 to $1,400 per month is hardly adequate reimbursement. However, it may be beneficial to advertise through the county Medical Society or to contact local physicians known to have an interest in geriatrics to see if they might be interested and qualified to assume the role. Also, if the facility is near an academic hospital with a geriatrics department, staff members there may be willing to apply for the position. Hiring the best possible physician for the role should be the objective of the nursing home administrator in consultation with the director of nursing. The American Medical Director's Association (AMDA), with its program of Certified Medical Directors, has helped to improve the level of training and awareness of physicians. The AMDA's current policy on the role and responsibilities of the medical director in a nursing home appears at the end of this chapter (see Figure 9.1).

An outstanding medical director can be a vital force in the facility's creation of a

(continued on p. 55)

The physician medical director should:

1. Exercise medical and clinical leadership in an interdisciplinary approach to resident care and care planning within the long-term care setting and interact with the attending staff as a colleague and a peer.

2. In collaboration with the nursing director, the administrator, and other health professionals, develop formal resident care policies for the facility that
   - provide for the total medical and psychological needs of the resident, including admission, transfer, discharge planning, range of services available to residents, emergency procedures, and frequency of physician visits in accordance with resident needs;
   - help enhance resident's rights as identified in the federally mandated Patient Bill of Rights;
   - show that these resident care policies are carried out, as reflected and documented in the minutes of the drug regimen review and quality assurance committees of the institution; and
   - include written designation of a registered nurse (with the guidance of the medical director as an advisory physician) as responsible for the day-to-day execution of these policies.

3. Perform the following roles with respect to resident care: (a) act as liaison with and coordinate the activities of other health professionals for the care of the resident; (b) in an emergency, be prepared to assume temporary responsibilities for the care of a resident, in the event that the resident's own attending physician or the designated alternate physician is not available.

4. Maintain a thorough knowledge of the federal, state, and local regulations and codes applicable to long-term care facilities, applicable standards of the Joint Commission on Accreditation of Healthcare Organizations, as well as the professional service and administrative requirements and expectations of participating public and private reimbursement programs.

5. Develop, amend, recommend, and implement appropriate clinical practices and medical care policies, with the cooperation and collaboration of health professionals and administrators within the long-term care institution, which include a way to ensure that each resident's medical regime is incorporated appropriately into the plan of care.

6. Act as the spokesperson of the medical staff (analogous to the chief-of-staff within a hospital), in cooperation with the administration and with the approval of the governing body, to develop rules, regulations, and policies for individual attending physicians who admit their patients to the facility.

FIGURE 9.1   The American Medical Directors' Association's policy on the role and responsibilities of the medical director in the nursing home.*

*Adopted as policy by AMDA December 1991.

7. Monitor the activities of attending physicians and intervene as needed on behalf of residents or the administration of the facility.
8. Review recommendations and reports of drug regimen review and quality assurance committees and take appropriate and timely action as needed to implement recommendations.
9. Routinely meet with nursing and other professional staff to discuss administrative, dietary, housekeeping issues, specific resident care problems, and professional staff needs for education or consultants, offering solutions to problems and identifying areas where policy should be developed.
10. Actively help develop ongoing in-service education programs for attending physicians and professional staff within the institution, in cooperation with the director of nursing and the administrator.
11. Act as a resource on resident care, new treatment modalities, and the pathophysiology of illness.
12. Obtain the services of qualified professionals to serve as consultants to several areas of special resident need, such as dentistry, podiatry, dermatology, and orthopedics.
13. Prepare a regular report summarizing his or her actions, concerns, and recommendations as medical director.
14. Represent the facility in discussions and meetings with other institutions on issues relevant to medical care.
15. Conduct an ongoing program for the evaluation and management of the health of the facility's employees, by (a) establishing policy and procedures, and (b) direct physical examination of employees, emphasizing freedom from significant infection, preemployment physical examinations and reexaminations, and compliance with local and state health regulations.
16. Help the facility administrator to ensure a safe and sanitary environment for residents and personnel, including review of incidents and accidents, identification of hazards to health and safety, and advice about possible correction or improvement of the environment.
17. Assist management in its review and response to any official medical review by federal, state, or local surveys and inspections.

FIGURE 9.1   (continued)

set of bylaws by which to organize the medical staff. Appendix A at the end of this book lists a model set of bylaws that can aid in achieving the goal of an effective organizational structure. The bylaws can also assist in the development of an application for clinical privileges, now required for accreditation by the Joint Commission on Accreditation of Healthcare Organizations (JCAHO).

The medical director should be personally involved in reviewing the credentials and privileges requested by all applicants to the medical staff. These clinical privileges should be maintained in an organized file and contain at least the following information:

- Copy of current license to practice medicine or other specialty
- Copy of current Federal Drug Enforcement Agency registration and state narcotics registration (if available in the state) when applicable
- List of clinical privileges the applicant is requesting from the facility
- Proof of current local hospital staff membership (this will allow the facility to forgo a formal review of the applicant in the National Data Bank since this will have been done by the hospital)
- Proof of current malpractice insurance (minimums may vary from state to state)
- Current resume/curriculum vitae listing educational background
- List of covering physicians and their telephone numbers

For physicians without current hospital staff membership, a formal review of their file and credentials can usually be obtained from the state Medical Society for a fee. All credentialing information and requests for clinical privileges should be kept strictly confidential at all times.

Appendix B shows a model application for clinical privileges that can be used to review the credentials of all licensed professionals wishing to work in a nursing home facility. This application can also be adapted to include the review of credentials for all health care professionals working within the facility.

Ideally, the medical director should meet weekly with the director of nursing to review the clinical events and any problems that developed within the past week. The director should also speak with staff members to be updated on events that have occurred since his or her last visit. Subsequently, the director of nursing should review with the medical director any of the following:

- clinical issues of importance involving other attending physicians' residents within the facility
- issues pertaining to JCAHO or state regulations
- nursing or personnel issues of note
- current safety issues (leaking roofs, broken equipment, construction, etc.)
- epidemics present in the facility
- elopements of residents from the facility that occurred since the last visit
- alleged resident abuse complaints

Safety issues and epidemics require the medical director's notification and involvement as clinically indicated by the situation. A record of all visits by the medical director to the facility should be maintained and kept at the facility. This log could include such items as issues discussed during that visit and any residents seen, although this is not required by regulation in most states.

The medical director serves on the medical board of the facility and often will be a member of the pharmacy and quality assurance committees. The medical director is also charged with officially reviewing incident reports as they occur in the facility and commenting to the medical board on any areas where intervention might be indicated based on his or her review of these reports.

The medical director has authority to sign monthly order summaries and to see another physician's patients in an emergency when the regular attending physician or covering physician is not available. However, it is imperative that if monthly orders are to be signed for another physician (due to that physician being overdue in his or her renewals), the resident be examined by the medical director and the orders checked for appropriateness and accuracy prior to signing them. Once the medical director's signature is on the monthly order renewal sheet, he or she is assuming liability for all the orders and medications listed. Additionally, a progress note should be written for any resident being seen by the medical director. Before a covering physician initiates therapy with any new antipsychotic agent on a resident, the medical history should be fully reviewed and the resident examined. Communication with family members may also be indicated.

Ideally, the medical director should be involved with employee health issues, including the annual physical examination of employees, emphasizing freedom from significant infection and compliance with all local and state health regulations regarding employment. Also, the medical director may be able to actively participate in the facility's ongoing in-service program, with special reference to employee health and safety issues.

Facility malpractice insurance covers the clinical activities of the medical director while he or she is acting in that role (i.e., for all emergency clinical duties of a medical director regarding residents for whom he or she is not the attending physician of record and for whom he or she does not routinely cross-cover for another physician). It is recommended that the medical director call the regular attending physician of any resident whom he or she sees in an emergency situation to allow for appropriate follow-up. In some instances, such as an acute medical emergency, it may be necessary to call the family as well.

If the director of nursing feels comfortable with the support the medical director is providing to the facility, he or she may be inclined to communicate problems that can arise within a facility and enlist the medical director's help in formulating solutions. Any person who is being screened for possible admission and has complex medical issues should also be reviewed by the medical director for appropriateness and to assist the facility in determining if the staff can meet the *total* care needs of this person. If the facility cannot meet the needs, then the medical director should support the facility in declining the request for admission. Additionally, all policies that relate to the medical care being rendered in the facility should be reviewed by the medical director for comments and suggestions.

During inspections, the medical director should be available to surveyors and staff, since his or her presence can be critical in many instances in obtaining a fair review process. If not physically present, he or she should be available by telephone for both the nursing home administrator and the director of nursing. While it is true that generally most surveyors will not seek out the medical director, the availability of the medical director to answer medical care questions that may arise during the survey process is very important. The medical director can also assist the facility in preparing for surveys by auditing a certain percentage of the charts and by identifying those with omitted signatures, overdue physical exams, or missing progress notes. These audits should be done routinely and are required annually under OBRA guidelines for at least 10% of the charts. If the medical director can be present during the exit conference, he or she may be in a better position to assist the facility in preparing answers to any deficiencies cited by the surveyors.

The medical director should work in conjunction with the director of nursing to facilitate the provision of the highest level of care possible within the facility. This includes communicating with attending physicians if it appears that

- Recommendations of consultants are not being followed up on or written documentation provided on why they were not being followed
- Monthly orders are not being signed in a timely manner
- Telephone calls from the nursing home are not being promptly answered by the attending or covering physician
- Progress notes during physician visits are not being written per the required federal/state regulations
- Residents admitted are not being seen within the prescribed 48- to 72-hour time frame
- Specialized services (e.g., intravenous therapy) are not being properly renewed or supervised
- Physician coverage arrangements are not adequate for the clinical needs of the residents residing in the facility
- Specialized units (e.g., subacute units without a separate medical director) are not receiving proper medical coverage
- Indicated medical, surgical, or other consultations are not being obtained

If properly selected, a medical director can be a valuable asset to the facility, aiding in the delivery of high-quality care to the residents. Every effort should be made to select the proper person for this vital position and integrate him or her into the decision-making process whenever medical issues are involved.

ADDITIONAL READINGS

Birn SW. The role of nursing home medical directors in successful survey outcomes. *Nursing Home Med.* 1995; 3:166–177.

Levenson SA. The new OBRA Enforcement Rule: Implications for attending physicians and medical directors (Parts I–V). *Nursing Home Med.* 1995; 3:3–7.

Weinberg AD. The medical director's role in disciplining attending physicians at nursing homes. *Journal of Medical Direction.* 1991; 1:24–30.

10 Tips From This Chapter
1. Screen for the best possible candidate for the position of medical director.
2. Have the director of nursing meet weekly with the medical director, and document these rounds in a log book.
3. A potential resident who appears to have a high acuity of care needs and for whom proper staffing may not be available should be screened by the medical director to ascertain whether admission to the facility is in the resident's best interest.
4. For any resident seen by the medical director, proper documentation should be maintained and notification of the primary physician should be given.
5. Immediately notify the medical director of all alleged abuse incidents, facility epidemics, or safety issues.
6. Incorporate the medical director in the in-service program of the facility.
7. The medical director should serve as the official liaison between the administration and attending physician staff when questions of appropriate medical care or coverage issues arise.
8. The medical director should oversee any clinical problems that may develop in the management of specialized units (e.g., subacute units) if a separate medical director is not appointed for that role.
9. The medical director should perform an annual audit of at least 10% of a facility's charts to ascertain that medical notes, orders, and required physical exams are being done on a timely basis.
10. The medical director should assist in preparing for all surveys and in helping to answer any questions raised on the delivery of medical care in the facility.

10

Legal Aspects of Risk Management

Lawsuits against nursing homes may involve both civil and professional (malpractice) areas. Environmental negligence is the term used for problems that involve the physical plant of the long-term care facility and that can result in injuries caused by slips or falls (usually on a wet floor), security breakdowns (e.g., theft), fires with associated injuries and/or loss of property, failure of equipment (e.g., scalding water from the breakdown of a regulator, broken wheelchairs, hazardous electrical appliances, or malfunctioning beds that lead to injury), or problems in areas of a facility that are undergoing repair (e.g., broken glass not repaired or cordoned off properly).[1] Professional negligence (malpractice) is a more complex problem and results in claims against attending physicians, the nursing staff, and the facility. It can include claims related to falls (with the resident either attended or unattended); medication errors; burns; untreated or undiagnosed infections, dehydration, mental status changes and allergic reactions to medications; improper discharge and/or transfer; and the development of pressure sores. Claims of negligence against nursing facilities can also involve the assault of one resident by another or by an intruder, staff abuse of residents, and the wandering of a resident away from the facility with subsequent injuries and violation of a resident's rights, such as the failure to obtain informed consent for specified treatments, participation in research projects, or medications.[2,3–6]

Presently, falls and related injuries account for two-thirds of all claims filed against nursing homes.[7] The other primary areas of claims include wandering-related injuries, neglect of a medical condition (especially pressure sores), environmental negligence, malfunctioning of equipment, and abuse of residents.[8] Resident abuse is a major area of concern of the public and consumer groups and is often highlighted on television exposé programs. Such abuse can be physical, restraint-related, or psychological.

The majority of lawsuits involving nursing homes are initiated by the family of the resident, rather than by the resident. Efforts to maintain a friendly relationship with residents and their relatives, friends, or colleagues may be critical in the avoidance of legal action.[9,10] There are a number of legal bases for filing a suit, and most involve specific state statutes, federal Medicare Conditions of Participation, and regulations that affect participation in Medicaid programs. In situations in which family members do not visit regularly or at all, an acute decline or death of a relative in a nursing home may bring out significant guilt, which might subsequently be channeled into a lawsuit. The most effective way to avoid these problems is to have open and honest communication and to treat the families of residents as "friends" and not just clients.

DISCOVERY ACTIONS BY THE PLAINTIFF'S ATTORNEY AFTER A LAWSUIT HAS BEEN FILED

The attorney for the plaintiff will seek information ("discovery") from the attending physician and the nursing home facility to determine the extent of injury, type of evaluation and treatment ordered, laboratory results, clinical data obtained by nursing staff, and other documentation to support the potential lawsuit. All records obtained by legal request will undoubtedly be reviewed by a health care professional (nurse and/or physician) hired by the plaintiff's lawyer prior to any court action. The attorney will be looking for deviations from the appropriate standard of care, as delineated by federal and state statutes or regulations, nursing home policy manuals, the parent corporation's regulations for its subsidiary homes, and other general standards that could be discussed by expert witnesses.

The leading federal statute affecting nursing home issues is 42 U.S.C. § 1396r (1990 Supp.), a section covering Medicaid law, which mandates that nursing homes receiving Medicaid (Title XIX) reimbursement provide appropriate nursing, medical, and rehabilitative activities, as well as social services, in order that each resident "attain or maintain the highest practicable physical, mental and psychological well-being" at a facility.[11] This act states that all services provided must meet professional standards of quality. A plaintiff's attorney may obtain copies of the most recent survey of a facility from the state licensing agency to review deficiencies cited by the inspectors.

Usual targets of discovery include time cards of the staff (not just schedules) to determine whether legal staffing minimums were maintained at all times. An attorney may look for any entries in the resident's record that were supposedly made by an employee when he or she was not clocked in as being present at work that day. A request may be made for all relevant nursing notes, resident care plans, incident reports, names and addresses of all employees who have left employment since the time in question, flow sheets, medication/general orders, in-service manuals, facility policy books, and any log books of the medical director. Efforts will be made to discover discrepancies between physician orders and documentation of compliance, resident care plans and actual care given, problems with fluid or food intake, or inconsistent documentation by nursing. Additionally, a search will be made for errors or omissions on charts, failure to inform the attending physician, chart entries made long after a particular incident occurred, and failure to update or follow resident care plans. Because of this, the medical director should inform staff that no editing or additions to any portion of a medical chart should be made without proper dating and labeling of such entries or changes.

Although the medical director may have no firsthand knowledge of the incident in question, he or she can be asked by the plaintiff's attorney to give a deposition if it appears that he or she should have had knowledge of the incident as it occurred and could have intervened as part of their responsibility for the overall supervision of attending physicians admitting residents to the facility. For example, after a facility-wide epidemic, an attempt will be made to determine whether the medical director should have been more diligent in monitoring the evaluation and treatment of affected individuals by the attending physician and whether he or she should have directly intervened in those cases where problems clearly existed. Testimony by the medical director could reveal confusion or poor communication on the part of the facility, which might aid the plaintiff's lawsuit. Since a medical director is covered by the facility's malpractice carrier (as an "also named" individual), the attorney assigned to defend the physician will also be defending the nursing home. The medical director may also retain private counsel at his or her own expense.

The initial contact that staff will have with the attorney for the plaintiff will usually be at a deposition. At the deposition numerous questions will be asked regarding the alleged incident or set of incidents. The individual being deposed will be sworn in and a court reporter will transcribe the testimony. Some questions will relate to the educational and professional background of the person being deposed. The attorney representing the nursing home will be present and can object to questions he or she feels are inappropriate. After the objection is raised for the record, the individual being deposed will be allowed to answer the question to the best of his or her ability. It is important to stress that if the individual does not remember a specific incident, he or she should say so and never guess. If the individual does not recall a particular document he or she supposedly signed, the plaintiff's attorney should be asked to produce the document for review. The individual should answer the question being asked and not what he or she thinks the attorney meant to ask. The defense attorney will also have the opportunity to ask questions. Any lack of cooperation or compliance on the part of the resident, especially as documented in the medical record, should be mentioned. The specific reason for any noted lack of cooperation or compliance should be documented by staff in the record (e.g., language barriers, hearing deficits, dementia, or acute medical illness with delirium).

After the deposition is concluded, the individual will be asked whether he or she wish to "read" (i.e., read the testimony after it is typed up) or "waive" (accept the typed report without review). Most prefer to review the testimony prior to signing it.

Many law firms make it standard practice to locate and interview former employees, looking for those who resigned due to what was perceived on their part as "poor care" or as an "unresponsive" director of nursing or administrator. These former employees can be particularly useful to potential plaintiffs. As a general rule, facilities need to monitor the attitude their staff has toward the institution as a whole. Methods of attaining this goal include the following:

1. Always interview all departing employees to ascertain any complaints or perceived weaknesses in the current administrative and nursing system. Promptly follow up on any identified problems.
2. Survey, on a regular basis, current employees to identify perceived problem areas and assign a staff member to investigate and make recommendations to the director of nursing and the administrator regarding possible solutions.
3. Create an orientation program for new employees that emphasizes the delivery of quality care and specific mechanisms on reporting suggestions or observed weaknesses to the appropriate responsible individual.
4. Provide ongoing in-service programs that cover conflict resolution and improving communication skills.
5. Instruct all supervisors to provide easy approachability by employees and a willingness to work with all staff members to improve the work environment and provide quality care. Include all licensed personnel and nursing assistants in the care-planning decisions and organized feedback sessions.
6. Instruct scheduling personnel to rotate difficult assignments for both nursing assistants and licensed personnel to avoid staff burnout and subsequent potential delivery of poor care.
7. Develop ways to encourage employees to submit innovative ideas on improving the delivery of care or to identify weaknesses in the current system with possible solutions.

Other potential witnesses include nursing students, visitors, and attending physicians. It is best not to view them as just "disgruntled former employees" or "outsiders," as their testimony is often used to corroborate certain gaps in the nursing home chart or the testimony of other key, directly involved individuals. In certain instances, the attending physician and/or the medical director will also be named in the lawsuit, depending on the alleged complaints. Neither should discuss the pending lawsuit in any manner with potential witnesses, whether they work in the facility or not. The attorney assigned to represent the nursing home will review the usual rules regarding pretrial actions and restrictions.

Expert affidavits by both nurses and physicians, based on their review of the nursing home chart, will also be obtained by the plaintiff attorney and used in any negotiations and/or trial. A sample medical affidavit is shown in Figure 10.1. These experts will provide the legal basis for any claims being alleged against the nursing

(continued on p. 68)

IN THE CIRCUIT COURT OF THE THIRTEENTH JUDICIAL CIRCUIT
IN AND FOR HILLSBOROUGH COUNTY, FLORIDA,
CIVIL DIVISION

Plaintiff,   Case number: 94-1034
Reginald Brown   Division: A

vs.

Hollow Grove Nursing Home
John A. Rivers, M.D., Attending Physician
Peter Wright, M.D., Medical Director

Defendants.

STATE OF FLORIDA

COUNTY OF HILLSBOROUGH:

Now comes Robert M. Green, M.D., being first duly cautioned and sworn, who deposes and says as follows:

1. My curriculum vitae, attached hereto as Exhibit A, accurately reflects my education, my training, and my experience as a physician experienced in the care and treatment of nursing home residents.
2. I have been trained and have experience in caring for nursing home residents in cooperation with registered nurses, licensed practical nurses, certified nursing assistants, and unlicensed nursing home personnel.
3. I have reviewed the following medical records and charts concerning REGINALD BROWN:

FIGURE 10.1 Sample affidavit of an expert physician regarding a nursing home malpractice case.

Note: Names and places have been changed. No similarity to any person, place, or incident is intended, and any such occurrence is purely coincidental.

a.	Big Valley Hospital:	8/13/90–7/09/91;
b.	Hollow Grove Nursing Home:	7/09/91–8/01/91;
c.	St. John's Hospital:	8/01/91–8/16/91;
d.	Hollow Grove Nursing Home:	8/16/91–6/19/92;
e.	St. John's Hospital:	6/19/92–7/03/92;
f.	Medicenter:	7/03/92–7/07/92;
g.	St. John's Hospital:	7/07/92–7/24/92;
h.	Medicenter:	7/24/92–8/12/92;

4. These records indicate a complete failure by the staff of HOLLOW GROVE NURSING HOME to conduct a nutritional or dietary evaluation necessary to implement a nutritional care plan suited to meet REGINALD BROWN's dietary needs in the least intrusive manner possible.

a. REGINALD BROWN had a nasogastric feeding tube inserted immediately upon return from St. John's Hospital on 8/16/91. The staff of HOLLOW GROVE NURSING HOME, particularly the care plan team, subsequently failed to perform blood work and conduct tests to determine REGINALD BROWN's appropriate calorie count. Furthermore, they failed to take the necessary steps to put him on a feeding program that would provide his nutritional requirements via a method less intrusive than the nasogastric tube.

b. The nasogastric tube is fed through the nose to the stomach. It is extremely uncomfortable and intrusive. REGINALD BROWN pulled the tube out numerous times and as a result had to be physically restrained during the majority of his stay at HOLLOW GROVE NURSING HOME.

c. From 4/1/91–4/12/91 a swallowing assessment was allegedly performed on REGINALD BROWN. The therapist recommended that a gastric or PEG tube (inserted directly into the stomach) be used over the more intrusive nasogastric tube.

d. Despite the recommendation from the therapist, HOLLOW GROVE NURSING HOME failed to replace the nasogastric tube with a less intrusive method of feeding. REGINALD BROWN was fed by the nasogastric tube and kept in restraints until his departure from HOLLOW GROVE NURSING HOME on 6/19/92.

e. It is my opinion that the continuing pattern of conduct of HOLLOW GROVE NURSING HOME's staff from August 16, 1991, to June 19, 1992, demonstrates a conscious and reckless indifference to REGINALD BROWN's health and rights, thereby depriving him of his right to adequate and appropriate health care and protective and supportive services. Such outrageous conduct constitutes abuse and neglect.

FIGURE 10.1   (continued)

5. The records from HOLLOW GROVE NURSING HOME indicate that the staff failed to provide REGINALD BROWN with adequate, appropriate, and timely medical care and at times were entirely inattentive to his medical needs.

a. A key example of this is the treatment of REGINALD BROWN in the latter half of July, 1991. During this time, REGINALD BROWN began to exhibit high temperatures and newly acquired pressure ulcers. The doctor was not notified of these significant changes until the morning of July 16, and he ordered more fluid for REGINALD BROWN. Twelve hours later REGINALD BROWN'S temperature was still high at 102° and the doctor was not notified. At 9:00 A.M. on July 17, his temperature was still 102° and at 2:00 P.M. it was 100.6°. At 9:00 P.M., REGINALD BROWN's family was concerned because he was not verbalizing and at midnight his temperature remained high at 101°. During July 18, REGINALD BROWN'S family was notified of his condition. However, the HOLLOW GROVE NURSING HOME staff had yet to notify the doctor that REGINALD BROWN was not responding to his July 16 order for fluids. Finally around 12 noon on July 19, after recording a temperature of 101.6°, the staff contacted the doctor and antibiotics were prescribed for REGINALD BROWN.

b. REGINALD BROWN's illness continued until it culminated on the morning of August 1, 1991, with a 104° temperature at 6:00 A.M. The doctor was not notified until 10:45 A.M. The staff of HOLLOW GROVE NURSING HOME act as the eyes and the ears for the physician. They have the primary responsibility of keeping the physician aware of any changes in the resident's condition and then to inform the doctor as to whether the order produced its intended results.

c. In my opinion the staff of HOLLOW GROVE NURSING HOME should have made the doctor aware of REGINALD BROWN's illness with the first significant change in his condition on July 15, 1992. Certainly, they should have notified him on the evening of July 16, 1992, when his order for fluids failed to bring about a positive change in REGINALD BROWN's condition. It was a clear example of neglect when the staff waited until 12 noon on July 19, 1991, to inform the doctor of REGINALD BROWN's unchanged condition.

d. It should be universally known by every licensed staff member of a nursing home that the presence of a temperature of 104° in a resident is a clear indication of a medical emergency requiring the immediate attention of a medical doctor. The near five-hour delay of the HOLLOW GROVE NURSING HOME's staff in notifying the doctor of REGINALD BROWN's condition on August 1, 1991, demonstrates their utter lack of attentiveness to his medical needs and their complete failure to render adequate, appropriate, and timely medical treatment.

e. It is my opinion that John A. Rivers, M.D., the attending physician for this resident, should have been able to detect through review of the record, examina-

FIGURE 10.1 (continued)

tion of the resident, and in discussions with nursing staff the poor care being rendered to this resident. He failed to do this and order appropriate interventions. It is further asserted that Peter Wright, M.D., the medical director, had a duty to review the care being rendered by both the facility and Dr. Rivers, which he failed to do and thus breached his agreement to provide these services.

6. HOLLOW GROVE NURSING HOME's failure to take steps to prevent the formation of pressure ulcers, and their inadequate and inappropriate treatment of the ulcers after their development, are the clearest examples of neglect rising to the level of abuse.

a. All licensed nursing home personnel should know that when a resident suffers a stroke, like REGINALD BROWN, with residual partial paralysis, they become susceptible to the formation of pressure ulcers. Furthermore, it is well known that such individuals require special attention and preventive measures to stave off the formation of pressure ulcers.

b. In my opinion, given the proper treatment, REGINALD BROWN could have remained free of pressure ulcers. The fact that he developed serious ulcers on his coccyx, hip, and left heel is evidence of HOLLOW GROVE NURSING HOME's staff's, especially the care plan team's, failure to implement reasonable and effective pressure-relieving measures.

c. To allow REGINALD BROWN's left heel to become gangrenous to the point of requiring amputation, despite the presence of foul-smelling drainage more than three weeks prior to his admission to the hospital, raises such neglect to the level of abuse.

7. It is further my opinion that the staff of HOLLOW GROVE NURSING HOME exploited REGINALD BROWN for financial gain. I reach this conclusion based upon the swallowing, speech, and physical therapy given to REGINALD BROWN in July 1991 and April 1992.

a. The therapists' notes describe REGINALD BROWN as being active in group activities and having the ability to wheel himself in a wheelchair. This is a direct contradiction of the nursing notes and minimum data set, which describe REGINALD BROWN as lacking cognitive and physical abilities and requiring total nursing care.

b. Furthermore, the therapies were allegedly administered during times when the nursing notes describe REGINALD BROWN as being very ill with high fevers. Swallowing therapy was allegedly conducted during a period when the nursing notes indicate he was being fed with a nasogastric tube going in his nose and down his throat.

8. The conduct by HOLLOW GROVE NURSING HOME and its staff described above causes me to conclude that no one at HOLLOW GROVE NURSING HOME was coordinating and overseeing REGINALD BROWN's care. This

FIGURE 10.1   (continued)

lack of coordination and oversight resulted in haphazard care and repeated instances of inexcusable neglect and abuse.

9. In addition, the conduct of HOLLOW GROVE NURSING HOME as set forth above displays a conscious indifference and reckless disregard for the rights, health, and safety of REGINALD BROWN.

10. All the opinions stated in this affidavit are expressed within a reasonable degree of medical probability and are based upon my education, training, experience, and review of the records listed in this affidavit.

11. This affidavit is not intended to, and does not, contain all of the opinions that I have reached concerning REGINALD BROWN's care at HOLLOW GROVE NURSING HOME.

Further, affiant sayeth naught.

ROBERT M. GREEN, M.D.

FIGURE 10.1   (continued)

home staff, the medical director, and/or the attending physician of a facility and will be available to testify at the trial.

If the case is not resolved through negotiations and comes to trial, the defense attorney provided by the nursing home malpractice carrier will review all standard procedures and anticipated areas of questioning he or she expects to be asked of any of the witnesses during the trial. Those involved should discuss any concerns or questions they may have at that time.[12]

The stress of any potential lawsuit is great, and it may take years for a case to actually be resolved. Not all requests for information from a nursing facility or physician's office or the taking of depositions result in a subsequent case; however, many do. Many of the more obvious cases where serious injury has resulted or negligence is admitted by one party will often be settled out of court. Because many cases reaching trial often result in jury awards to the plaintiff in the millions of dollars, usually only the most defensible cases actually ever end up in a courtroom. Good documentation, the delivery of quality care, the maintenance of high staff morale, and effective communication skills are necessary to minimize the possibility of any legal action being filed against the staff and/or the facility.

REFERENCES

1. Annotation: Hospital's liability to patient for injuries sustained from defective equipment furnished by hospital for use in diagnosis or treatment of patient. *Am Law Reports.* 33d 1967; 14:1254–1261.

2. Kapp MB. Risk management: Preventing malpractice suits in long term care facilities. *QRB*. 1986; 12:109–113.

3. Weinberg AD, Pals JK, Levesque PG, et al. Dehydration and death during febrile episodes in the nursing home. *JAGS*. 1994; 42:968–971.

4. Waxman HM, Klein M, Carner EA. Drug misuse in nursing homes: An institutional addiction? *Hosp Community Psychiatry.* 1985; 36:886–887.

5. Annas G. "Transfer trauma" and the right to a hearing. *Hastings Cent Rep.* 1980; 10:23–24.

6. Garibaldi R, Brodine S, Matsumiya S. Infections among patients in nursing homes. *NEJM*. 1981; 305:731–735.

7. Fraser MR. Nursing home civil litigation. *Nursing Home Medicine*. 1995; 3:79–82.

8. Micheletti J, Shlala T. Integrating risk management and quality assurance programs. *Contemporary LTC*. 1988; 11:79–83.

9. Hall RE. Doctor-patient rapport: Key to avoiding a malpractice suit. *Physician's Management*. 1983; 23:120–126.

10. Sommers PA. Malpractice risk and patient relations. *J Nat Med Assoc*. 1984; 76:953–956.

11. 42 U.S.C.A. § 1396r (b)(2) (West Supp 1990).

12. Mandell M. What to expect from your malpractice attorney. *A J Nursing*. 1995; Nov: 29–31.

10 Tips From This Chapter

1. Falls and related injuries account for two-thirds of all claims filed against nursing homes. Pay special attention to fall prevention programs in the nursing home.

2. Pressure ulcer assessment, treatment, and monitoring should be a priority of a facility's risk management program.

3. Medical directors should be informed of all significant events occurring in the facility at least on a weekly basis.

4. Efforts to maintain a friendly relationship with nursing home residents and their relatives, friends, or colleagues may be critical in avoiding legal action.

5. Do not discuss a pending lawsuit with any potential witnesses. If you have any questions, contact the attorney assigned to represent you.

6. Provide ongoing in-service programs on conflict resolution, communication skills, and risk management techniques.

7. Survey, on a regular basis, current employees to identify perceived problem areas.

8. Train supervisors to provide easy approachability by all employees and a willingness to work with staff members to improve the work environment.

9. Develop ways to provide positive reinforcement for employees who submit innovative ideas on improving the delivery of care or identifying weaknesses in the current system.

10. The maintenance of good documentation, the delivery of quality care, and the development of effective communication skills should be emphasized with all staff members.

11

Creating and Implementing an Effective Risk Management Program

Risk management in long-term care can best be defined as a "facility-wide program designed to reduce preventable injuries and accidents and to minimize the financial severity of any claims" that involve residents of LTC facilities.[1,2,3] The bottom line, however, of any program is to foster those policies and procedures that aim to improve overall quality of care for residents living within that facility. Effective management requires the identification of high-risk areas and procedures and the implementation of corrective or preventive actions throughout a facility. Many LTC facilities have already developed extensive mechanisms for continuous quality improvement and reviews of utilization, which include the use of self-appraisal guides,[4] in an effort to minimize injuries to residents, improve quality of care, and diminish or eliminate any resulting potential legal liability.

Under the new standards detailed in the Omnibus Budget Reconciliation Act (OBRA) of 1987 (and subsequent revisions), in conjunction with existing state regulations, medical directors of facilities have increased responsibility for monitoring the standard of care delivered by all attending physicians and consultants at each facility. It is important that they acquire an attitude of mutual support, with feedback to nursing staff and administration, and the ability to recognize and treat potential and actual problems within the facilities.[5,6] However, they are not given any specific authoritative powers under OBRA to enforce these standards.

Attending physicians admitting persons to an LTC facility have a responsibility to provide care for their nursing home residents 365 days a year and to arrange suitable coverage during any absences. They must respond promptly to acute medical changes in their residents and institute appropriate therapy, which can include transfer to a hospital when indicated (Table 11.1). Appropriate evaluation and treatment are required for all fevers, falls, reactions to medications, nonresponses to ordered treatments, and abnormal laboratory results. The attending physician is also responsible for communicating to the family (in cases in which a resident is deemed incompetent) all significant changes in their relative's condition and to discuss treatment options and obtain informed consent (including do not resuscitate orders, feeding tube placement, and neuropsychoactive medications). For documentation purposes, progress notes must be written regularly (based on the required frequency of visits, usually every 30 to 60 days after the initial admission period). These notes must address any problems or illnesses that have occurred since the last visit. They also must address any ongoing medical issues, discharge planning, rehabilitation potential, nutrition and hydration status, functional status, continued need for restraints or neuropsychoactive medications, changes in cognitive function, and other psychosocial needs.

The nursing home has an obligation to provide a safe environment with appropriate nursing care (including specialized services such as physical therapy and intravenous therapy when indicated and appropriate), ongoing resident assessment, and the supervision of all allied health providers and nursing assistants in caring for the medical and psychosocial needs of all residents in the facility.

Nursing care plans should be modified as needed if the current interventions are not resolving the identified problem. For those facilities going to a "paperless" charting system, it is critical that all nursing assistants and other allied health providers be able to access the care plan without difficulty. Training needed to

TABLE 11.1 Responsibilities of the Attending Physician at a Nursing Home

- Respond in a timely manner to acute changes in each resident's condition and order appropriate intervention.
- Follow up on inadequate responses to previously initiated treatments or obvious complications, drug interactions, and side effects of all prescribed treatments.
- Follow all state and federal guidelines on required medical visits and interdisciplinary treatment planning.
- Respond in a timely manner to telephone inquiries from the nursing staff 24 hours a day.
- Provide alternate and appropriate coverage by another physician when unavailable to offer care for the residents.
- Discuss the condition and treatment options for legally incompetent residents with next of kin or a designated legal representative.
- Document all decisions related to do-not-resuscitate orders, neuropsychoactive medications, or physical restraints in the chart after appropriate discussions with the resident and/or a designated family member.
- Provide adequate and appropriate follow-up care for all abnormal laboratory results.

allow all staff members to become proficient in the use of a computer must be given prior to the initiation of a totally paperless system for the delivery and charting of care for any resident. This training should be well documented, and each staff member should be required to demonstrate competency in the computerized system. JCAHO regulations do not prohibit a paperless system but insist that all providers have access to the computerized health record and a specific electronic signature assigned only to that one individual.

RECOMMENDATIONS FOR EFFECTIVE RISK MANAGEMENT

Recommended procedures that all staff should follow include avoidance of negative comments in the resident's record (Table 11.2). Such comments not only erode morale among the staff but also prove detrimental during any legal action. Staff members who routinely write such negative comments should be counseled, or, if such comments are made by a physician, the facility's medical director should speak to him or her. Also, facilities might consider the establishment of "physician notification parameters" to alert nursing staff as to when to contact the attending physician, immediately or the next office day, depending on the urgency of the problem (Table 11.3). These parameters include such issues as bleeding, changes in mental status, chest pain, diarrheal disease, edema, emesis, feeding tube problems, falls, family questions and requests, medication errors, abnormal laboratory values, pressure sores, seizures, shortness of breath, skin rashes, changes in vital signs, and weight loss. Early intervention in acute illness often is the best method of preventing serious morbidity and mortality in this population.

TABLE 11.2 Maintenance of a Positive Medical Record by Staff

- *Avoid criticizing physicians or any staff member for written comments or actions taken by them in the care of a resident:*
    (e.g., "This incompetent nurse obviously didn't read my last note or she wouldn't have allowed Mrs. Y to get out of bed, fall, and break her hip.")
- *Avoid writing damaging comments that may have no basis in fact:*
    (e.g., "This resident's problem is entirely due to Nurse X's not doing her job.")
- *Physicians should not refuse to change medical orders just to "get back" at regulations viewed as "coercive" or "meddling":*
    (e.g., "During his regular review, the consultant pharmacist indicated that a serum digoxin level was recommended for this resident according to state guidelines. I'll be the one to decide if and when this test should be ordered, not a pharmacist!")

TABLE 11.3   Events That Require Immediate Notification of the
                 Physician

Clinical Trigger	*Immediate Response Required*
Acute bleeding	• Uncontrolled or repeated episodes • Bloody emesis, stool (nonhemorrhoidal), vaginal drainage, or urine
Change in mental status	• All acute changes in mental status or sleep-wake cycle from baseline
Chest pain	• New onset or recurrent pain not relieved in 10 minutes by previously ordered NTG (3 doses) • All chest pain with concurrent changes in vital signs, diaphoresis, vomiting, or shortness of breath
Diarrheal disease	• Acute onset with multiple stools, significant fluid loss, blood in stool, or any change in vital signs
Edema	• Acute onset in one leg • Acute onset with redness or tenderness • Edema concurrent with shortness of breath
Emesis	• Bloody or coffee-ground composition • Repeated episodes of vomiting with concurrent abdominal pain
Feeding tube problems	• Required for hydration/nutrition but nursing staff unable to replace tube in a timely manner • Excessive residuals
Falls	• All falls; mention any suspected injury when speaking with the attending physician • Change in mental status of a resident with a history of a recent fall within past 2 weeks
Family questions/requests	• The family demands to speak with the attending physician immediately about a relative

TABLE 11.3   (continued)

Clinical Trigger	*Immediate Response Required*
Medication errors	• All errors, whether or not symptoms are present currently
Abnormal laboratory values	• All laboratory "panic" values (unless results have been consistently at this level and the attending physician is aware of them), although these values may be modified by facility protocols or a specific physician's written order • Positive urine/sputum cultures ordered for work-up of an acute problem • PT/INRs for residents on warfarin which are outside of parameters ordered by the attending physician
Pressure sores	• Stage II, III, or IV if receiving no treatment, facility protocols not available, or no significant improvement from previous prescribed therapy • Stage I should be reported on the next business day or earlier if a treatment order is needed
Seizures	• All seizures, with or without a previous history
Shortness of breath	• New onset or with chest pain • Ashen, dusky, or cyanotic appearance • Labored breathing
Skin rashes	• Significant urticaria or swelling • Rash with or without difficulty breathing in any resident taking new medication
Changes in vital signs	• Any significant change in systolic blood pressure (≥ 180 mm Hg or ≤ 90 mm Hg) unless readings are constant and the attending physician is well aware of them; or a specific mm Hg change as ordered by the physician over the resident's baseline • Resting pulse ≥ 120 or ≤ 55 • Respiratory rate ≥ 26 or ≤ 10 • Temperature $\geq 100°$ oral (unless modified by facility protocols)

In-services and educational offerings for nursing staff are a critical component of all risk management programs and help to achieve quality control.[6] With the high turnover rate of staff in certain categories (e.g., nursing assistants) at many facilities, quarterly or other regular repetition may be needed. These programs may be presented by the supervisory staff, the consultant pharmacist, the medical director, or outside experts contracted to cover certain high-risk areas (e.g., falls, pressure sores, or resident abuse). After the educational process and relevant documentation have been completed, a follow-up program is essential to ensure optimal quality assurance in the nursing home. To this end, developing measurable criteria for use in the review of care should be developed, and a member of the staff should be designated to perform appropriate studies.[7]

Nursing notes should be clear and concise when they address a resident's problems. It could be useful to regularly schedule in-service programs on the proper writing of nursing progress notes to review the key items that should always be included in any note. For emergency situations, the nurse's progress notes (or the general progress note section, if combined) should document all attempts to contact the physician, family, or designated legal representative. Also, all physician orders and the subsequent response to ordered treatments should be recorded. Nursing staff should always contact the attending physician if the resident's condition worsens or fails to respond adequately to the ordered treatment.

A lapse in medical record documentation indicates, for legal purposes, that the ordered medical treatment or assessment was not done. Routine scheduled chart audits will detect discrepancies, and appropriate feedback can be given to staff members to avoid these problems in the future. Late entries, properly labeled, are the correct way to add to a record when such lapses are found.

Incident reports should be filed by staff for any significant incident occurring at the facility and may be filled out by any employee or consultant.[6] The medical director and director of nursing should be notified immediately of all major incidents, in particular, alleged charges of abuse. These incident reports should be reviewed by the Medical Board and any identifiable patterns thoroughly investigated in order to propose interventions to deal with any identified negative outcomes or high risk areas.

Some facilities have a type of report known as a report of a potentially compensable event (PCE). A PCE is defined as any departure from normal resident care or any accident that might result in an injury for which the LTC facility could be held legally and financially responsible. Indicators of potentially legal issues include problems due to misdiagnosis, improper treatment, pressure ulcers, epidemics, complaints of poor care, or unexpected deaths. Table 11.4 lists discrepancies, errors, and omissions in a medical chart that a plaintiff's attorney will look for to bolster any alleged malpractice claims. The inclusion of a computer program to monitor trends may be useful at larger facilities for identification of potential problem areas.

TABLE 11.4   Incidents and Indicators of Potential Legal Problems Associated With a Medical Record in a Long-Term Care Facility

- Missing charting or failure to record properly prescribed treatments
- Alterations and/or deletions of any entries
- Entries out of sequence
- Use of a restraint without an appropriate physician's order or documentation
- Treatment of pressure ulcers without a physician's order or any deviation from an order
- Failure to report abnormal results of blood analyses to the attending physician
- Use of neuropsychoactive medications without an appropriate order or documentation
- Errors in medication administration
- A change in a resident's condition, nutrition, or hydration status without notification of the attending physician
- Missing vital signs
- Absent or tardy weekly and/or monthly summaries
- Evidence of inadequate attention to the needs of the resident

All facilities should have an organized and systematic procedure for responding to identified problem areas within the facility and for addressing and correcting any faulty aspects of care or policy. Incident reports should be used by the facility to develop databases that allow an analysis of incidents in an effort to avoid future repetition of similar events and not as an adversarial type of punishment for problems reported by the staff.[8]

Recommendations

Listed below are recommendations for effective risk management within an LTC facility. These may need to be modified or expanded depending on each facility's particular needs and resident population.

1. Offer regular in-service presentations on risk management issues for all staff, scheduled to allow for attendance by personnel from all three shifts. These programs should not only present factual information (e.g., how to keep better records) but sensitize staff members to the interpersonal and communication components of risk management issues. They should also stress that a positive attitude toward residents and their families can go a long way to reducing the occurrence of potential legal action and improving relations with residents' relatives.

2. Establish a risk management committee with the administrator, the director of nursing, and the medical director as required members, in addition to other

appropriate staff. Always generate incident reports for all events and use these as a database to identify any specific patterns within the facility so that a corrective plan of action can be formulated. All significant findings should be reported to the medical board. The medical director can also use this committee to focus on those high-risk procedures and medications that may need further evaluation or follow-up by the attending physician.

3. Contact the family and attending physician concerning all critical incidents, changes in a resident's condition, or abnormal laboratory results (notify the covering doctor or the medical director if the primary attending physician is not available). Always investigate specific incidents of injury to residents and document any corrective action taken by the facility. Do not hide, disguise, change, or otherwise interfere with the proper evaluation and treatment of injuries sustained at the facility. Report all incidents to the proper authorities as legally required. Avoid, at all costs, any editing of the nursing home chart. Clearly document all late entries as such.

4. Members of a restraint committee should routinely monitor the continued need for, frequency of use, and method of application of all restraints used within a facility. They should do more than just simply check that a physician's order has been filed and that a progress note has been written to justify the continued use of the restraint, although these are also required.

5. Use family council meetings as a forum to build resident and family support for the facility. Such meetings may also be used to discuss areas of concern that arise. The medical director or another attending physician should be present, on a regular basis, for short discussions of specific problems, medical topics, or facility programs.

6. The medical director should be an active member of all major committees and should be involved early on in any complaints against an attending physician in cases of alleged resident abuse and in facilitywide epidemics. The medical director should act as a liaison with other attending physicians when communication or coverage issues are involved. He or she should also be comfortable in issuing emergency coverage orders in cases in which the primary attending physician cannot be readily located or when a facilitywide epidemic or other health risk exists. An ineffective medical director can be a serious handicap to an effective risk management program. All contracts should specify the exact number of hours of employment, responsibilities of the medical director, and administrative authority that he or she may use to monitor quality of care issues.

7. The director of nursing (or designee) should regularly review the assignments of nursing assistants to difficult or abusive residents within the facility to ensure that rotation of assignments occurs. This strategy will help to reduce staff burnout and the potential for staff-initiated abuse.

8. Pressure ulcers continue to be a major and highly visible risk management issue that needs to be attacked aggressively. Consider the formation of a "skin care team" that will routinely assess the skin condition of each new resident and will be responsible for overseeing and coordinating the evaluation, treatment, and fol-

low-up care of all pressure ulcers that develop within the facility. This team, in conjunction with physician input, may also wish to develop and implement standardized treatment protocols for all stages of pressure ulcers.

9. All complaints of alleged resident abuse should be taken seriously and investigated thoroughly. Just because a resident may be legally incompetent or have some degree of cognitive impairment does not mean the story being told is totally without merit. If some members of your staff have repeated claims of resident abuse against them, it is best to identify them early and to rotate their assignments or terminate their employment after appropriate investigation.

10. CQI programs in a facility should also be used to identify high-risk areas or procedures in a facility and the data collected used to formulate interventions and changes in policy, which can be effective in reducing this risk. Follow-up of implemented plans should be done to permit an objective review of these interventions. Two sample CQI plans are shown in Table 11.5 and Table 11.6.

11. Resident care plans should be adjusted if the current treatment is not improving the identified area for intervention. Prepackaged care plans should be used with caution, since they may not readily encourage independent thought and individualized input to a particular resident's care needs.

12. An effective risk management program requires the facility to foster a positive attitude toward problems and not an "us versus them" mentality. Responses to concerns must be enthusiastic with the aim of avoiding repetition, and not just for the purpose of minimizing potential liability or assignment of blame. All staff members need to be educated about the principles of mutual responsibility for preventing problems, addressing outcome issues, and formulating plans for the resolution of identified high-risk areas.

Risk management should be a major goal for the administration, physicians, nurses, consultants, and all those who work in the nursing home setting. With increases in regulatory processes and increased monitoring of resident outcomes, it is imperative not only to deliver the best possible care to nursing home residents but also to establish well-organized mechanisms for identifying potential problems and to develop plans to prevent or reduce repetitive occurrences. As always, teamwork will continue to play a critical role in any successful program.

TABLE 11.5   Sample CQI Plan # 1: Indicator Development Form

I. Nursing Service

II. Aspect of Care: INCIDENCE OF PRESSURE ULCERS

III. Indicator Statement
1. Early detection of pressure ulcers
2. Treatment plan by interdisciplinary team
3. Evaluation and reduction of underlying causes

IV. Definition of Terms
Pressure ulcer: any lesion caused by unrelieved pressure resulting in damage of underlying tissue over a bony prominence

Incidence: rate at which a certain event occurs, as the number of new cases of a specific entity occurring during a certain period

V. Rationale
Heighten awareness of skin care and reduce incidence of new pressure ulcers in the nursing home following admission

VI. Components of Quality Assessed by Indicator
- *Effectiveness* of care provided to residents in preventing pressure ulcers from occurring
- *Timeliness* in detection of pressure ulcer formation at an early stage

VII. Underlying Factors
- Comorbidity of multiple, chronic illnesses
- Contributing factors of immobility/limited activity levels, incontinence, and altered nutritional/hydration status

VIII. Threshold for Evaluation
- *Numerator* = number of events (pressure ulcers) occurring during the quarter being reviewed
  Denominator = entire resident population of the nursing home (to be determined at the end of the quarter being reviewed)
- Incidence rate: > 0%

IX. Data Collection
- Source: information collected by registered nurses. The staging of pressure ulcers used is consistent with the recommendations of the National

TABLE 11.5 (continued)

Pressure Ulcer Advisory Panel and is followed by the Agency for Health Care Policy and Research.
- Sample size: entire resident population of the nursing home
- Frequency: quarterly
- Type: concurrent

X. Responsibility: Nursing home staff members in conjunction with the CQI coordinator for Nursing Service

---

TABLE 11.6 Sample CQI Plan # 2: Indicator Development Form

I. Medical Service

II. Aspect of Care: DRUG UTILIZATION—NEUROPSYCHOACTIVE MEDICATIONS: Usage and possible reduction with proper documentation

III. Indicator Statement
1. Appropriate indication for use with stated medical diagnosis and/or targeted behavior to be managed in progress note
2. Documentation every six (6) months in the progress note of any evidence of drug dosage reduction or evidence of drug taper with possible discontinuance if clinically indicated

IV. Definition of Terms
Neuropsychoactive medication: exerting an effect on the mind or modifying mental activity

The antipsychotics being monitored under this CQI indicator which are available at this facility include the following:

chlorpromazine	fluphenazine	haloperidol
molindone	perphenazine	risperidone
trifluperazine	thioridazine	loxapine
thiothixene	clozapine	

V. Rationale
Maximize resident's functional potential and well-being while minimizing adverse reactions

TABLE 11.6   (continued)

VI. Components of Quality Assessed by Indicator
- *Appropriateness* of its prescription by specified diagnosis
- *Efficacy* and *safety* as evidenced by documentation in the progress notes on targeted behavior and possible reduction of dosage or discontinuance of medication if clinically indicated

VII. Underlying Factors
- Comorbidity with organic mental syndromes (e.g., dementia)—higher, prolonged dosing may be indicated as evidenced by the resident's response or clinical record

VIII. Threshold for Evaluation
- *Numerator* = number of cases (residents receiving antipsychotic medication therapy) not meeting the above indicators
  Denominator = at least 30 cases or, if less than that number, 100% of cases will be reviewed
- Clinical events: <100%

IX. Data Collection
- Source: chart review
- Sample size: at least 30 cases (residents receiving antipsychotic medication therapy) or, if less than that number, 100% of cases will be reviewed
- Frequency: quarterly
- Type: retrospective

X. Responsibility: CQI coordinator for Nursing Service/medical director

REFERENCES

1. Kapp MB. Risk management: Preventing malpractice suits in long term care facilities. *QRB*. 1986; 12:109–113.
2. Khonen RB, Jr. Liability: Suits against nursing homes seem to be on the upswing. *American Health Care Assoc J*. 1978; 4:36–37.
3. Duran GS. On the scene: Risk management in health care. *Nursing Admin Quarterly*. 1980; 5:19–36.
4. American Health Care Association (AHCA). *Quest for Quality: A Self-Appraisal Guide for Long Term Care Facilities*. Washington, DC: AHCA, 1982.
5. Levenson SA. The New OBRA enforcement rule: Implications for attending

physicians and medical directors. *Nursing Home Medicine.* 1995; 3:83–85, 3:122–126, 3:150–154.
6. Allen JE. Effective risk management in long-term care. *J of Long-Term Care Admin.* 1991; 19:43–46, 49.
7. Micheletti J, Shlala T. Integrating risk management and quality assurance programs. *Contemporary LTC.* 1988; 11:79–83.
8. Gurwitz JH, Sanchez-Cross M, Eckler MA, et al. The epidemiology of adverse and unexpected events in the long-term care setting. *JAGS.* 1994; 42:33–38.

---

10 Tips From This Chapter

1. Risk management programs require the support, participation, and interaction of *all* staff members.
2. Avoid any editing, additions, or deletions to the nursing home chart. Late entries should be properly labeled as such.
3. Notify the attending physician and family of all significant changes in a resident's condition.
4. Effective communication among staff, residents, and their families is critical in the successful implementation of any risk management program.
5. Nursing and nursing assistant assignments of difficult or heavy-care residents should be routinely rotated to avoid staff burnout.
6. All pressure ulcers should be aggressively evaluated, treated, and monitored in a systematic fashion.
7. Risk management–related lectures should be offered on a regular basis to staff of all shifts.
8. The medical director should be involved with all facility-wide epidemics or other health problems.
9. CQI programs should be used to identify high-risk areas or procedures and serve as the basis for the formation of intervention strategies.
10. Modify resident care plans if a particular treatment is ineffective in the resolution of an identified problem.

12

Risk Management in the 1990s and Beyond

Risk management remains an important and highly visible aspect of good long-term care management. Whereas, at this writing, most malpractice insurance rates for long-term care remain relatively low (less than $120 per bed per year in most states), this situation may change dramatically as large jury awards and settlements, resulting from poor quality care being delivered at long-term care facilities, continue to occur across the country. As has happened on the acute care side of health care delivery, such rising malpractice awards may increase mandated continuing educational requirements for health care providers set by the insurance companies as a precondition for continued coverage. Insurance providers may insist on specialized educational training in risk management for all nursing staff, medical directors, and attending physicians.

Education and communication will remain the key ingredients to reducing overall risk and providing quality care to residents in this setting. Educational in-service programs undoubtedly will need to broaden the subject areas covered and should be mandatory for all shifts. The expanded use of videotaping of these programs for later repetition may prove very useful in this context. Physicians, pharmacists, and other health care providers will also need to participate on a more regular basis in the educational activities of the nursing homes in which they attend.

Risk management, by its most basic definition, is concerned with providing quality care and responding to unexpected events in a positive manner to prevent future recurrence. It is not about writing incident reports mandated by state regulation or saving money to be more cost-effective at the expense of appropriate staffing levels. Although the ongoing treatment of chronic disease or acute illness occupies the vast majority of a nursing home staff's time, this setting can still be an ideal location to practice preventive care and interventions designed to prevent injuries to the residents, especially as they relate to falls. Administrators of effective risk management programs appreciate this fact and design their operations to truly provide individualized treatment and specialized services when indicated after appropriate evaluation.

Given the proliferation of federal and state regulations concerning the operation of long-term care facilities and the rising number of awards for malpractice in this area, it is clear that a written regulation does not guarantee that the care it specifies will necessarily be carried out. Quality care requires an involved and motivated staff, along with administration, and cannot be the province of just one department or one assigned staff member.

Having made these points, it is also obvious that for many of the nation's 19,000 nursing homes, economic considerations are not trivial concerns for the individual administrators. As salary lines consume the vast majority of nursing home budgets, cost containment often has the effect of limiting the number of staff present on evening and weekend shifts. However, if effective risk management is to be practiced, each facility must be mindful of the concept of total nursing care over the entire 24-hour period, 7 days a week. This would include the use of supervisory personnel on weekends and holidays during day and evening work tours, with on-call capability for night shifts. The residents being evaluated for potential admission to a facility will also need to have their total care requirements carefully reviewed *before* admission, not only by the admission's coordinator of the facility but by the attending physician and/or the medical director.

Increasing the number of physicians willing to take a more active role in providing long-term care coverage in their respective communities remains an elusive goal in most areas of the country. Nursing home medicine remains relatively unappealing to most doctors, and while reimbursement for such care has increased, it is often not in proportion to the 365-day-a-year coverage required.

Long-term care in the 1990s and into the new century is expected to rise to the highest levels ever as the majority of people requiring nursing home placement are in the over-85 age bracket. This group remains the largest growing portion of the U.S. population. The industry must be prepared to deliver consistent quality care if it is to survive further regulatory intrusions by state and federal actions and if it is to meet the expectations of clients and their families. If reimbursement issues become a crucial factor in providing required needs, political action may be needed to investigate and legislate improved ways of paying for such desired quality care. Also, as the Medicaid system undergoes change and reinvention, nursing homes may find themselves suddenly with decreasing state-funded revenues in the face of increasing medically complex residents that may subsequently lead to quality-of-care issues for many residents.

This book has covered the major areas that anyone concerned with risk management in long-term care will need to be familiar with in order to design and implement an appropriate and useful program. It is important to stress that a good risk management program requires a fluid, ongoing process that allows supervisors and staff to respond to new problems as they arise in a facility. It also cannot be carried out without the enthusiastic and unqualified support of the nursing home administrator and the director of nursing.

The next 10 years will bring major changes to the entire health care industry in this country, with or without federal health care reform, and long-term care will be one of the major components of a leaner, more efficient acute care system transferring more unstable patients to long-term care facilities. The U.S. public has a history of expecting the very best from its health care system, and the long-term care sector will be no exception to these high expectations. The establishment and expansion of risk management programs will undoubtedly become a key component of all long-term care facility operations in the near future.

13

Case Presentations and Question Review

CASE # 1*

An 82-year-old white male was admitted from home, where he had lived for the past 20 years, to Harbor Lights Nursing Home on 10/25/95. His medical record indicated he had been diagnosed in the past with probable Alzheimer's disease and hypertension. The primary reasons for admission to the nursing home were to provide assistance with activities of daily living and to maintain a better nutritional intake. A physician assistant (PA) examined the resident 5 days after admission and did not note any significant medical problems at that time. The admitting physical exam, performed by the attending physician 25 days after admission to the facility, revealed a BP of 140/80 with a pulse of 68 and, other than moderate cognitive impairment on neurological testing (oriented × 1 only), the rest of the exam was essentially within normal limits. The resident's only medication was Calan CD 240 mg once a day to control hypertension.

Summary of Events

1. The Minimum Data Set completed shortly after admission showed no risk factors for delirium or dehydration.
2. He was admitted on 10/25 but not seen until 5 days later by the PA. (The attending physician did not actually see the resident until 25 days later.)
3. The resident became slightly more confused and "agitated" according to the staff 4 days after admission. Over the telephone, an order from the attending physician was received for Ativan 1 mg 3 times a day and a request given that a

---

*All names and places have been changed to protect the confidentiality of this case.

psychiatric consultation be obtained. The psychiatrist saw the resident 3 days later and diagnosed in the chart:

- Senile dementia with delirium
- Adjustment reaction to facility

He recommended Buspar 5 mg 3 times a day for 7 days and then increased the dose to 10 mg 3 times a day. The Ativan was to be stopped only after the 10 mg of Buspar was started. The attending physician did not order any work-up of the acute delirium. The nursing home staff did not question him on this point.

4. Within 1 week after admission, it was noted that the resident's daily food/fluid intake was down to 50% to 60% of the total provided on the tray. This information was recorded in the nursing notes but not called to the attending physician's office. The resident appeared more confused and disoriented since receiving both the Buspar and Ativan concurrently.

5. Three weeks after admission the resident developed a fever of 100.1° F. However, this information was never called to the attending physician's attention. The resident subsequently became extremely agitated and confused, and a new telephone order from the PA for Mellaril 10 mg 3 times a day and Haldol 5 mg IM stat was received by the nursing staff for these complaints.

6. The attending physician, making his first visit to the resident 4 weeks after admission, apparently did not review the extensive nursing notes detailing the change in mental status and decline in food consumption, as he made no comment regarding these clinical issues in his note. Also, he apparently did not review the psychiatric consultation note in the chart, as his entire progress note read as follows: "Chart reviewed, pt. examined, treatment and diagnoses reviewed."

7. Five weeks after admission, the resident was found to be quite lethargic. An order to hold the Mellaril was finally obtained by the nursing staff. Approximately 48 hours later the resident appeared extremely dehydrated, confused, and almost totally unresponsive. The attending physician was called and an order given to send the resident to the local hospital emergency department for evaluation. Despite intensive rehydration interventions, this resident died several days later. A malpractice suit was subsequently instituted against the nursing home and attending physician. (See Table 13.1 for a review of laboratory data for both the LTC facility and the hospital.)

Discussion Questions

1. Does the estate of the plaintiff have a real complaint against the nursing home and the attending physician?
2. Where did the attending physician fail to intervene properly?
3. Where did the nursing home fail to intervene properly?
4. Could this suit have been avoided?

TABLE 13.1   Lab Data

10/28/95 (nursing home)	Na 142	Cl 108	BUN 19	Cr 0.9
11/28/95 (hospital emergency department)	Na 182*	Cl 141*	BUN 156*	Cr 3.2*
Admitting nursing home weight:	210 lbs.			
Hospital admitting weight:	180 lbs. (down 30 lbs.)			

* Markedly elevated values

5. Are telephone orders for major tranquilizers for residents with new or increasing agitation/combativeness relatively safe to give?
6. What is the proper role of a psychiatry consultant?

Comments

The four criteria that must be satisfied in order for a malpractice action to have merit are:

1. The named individual had an established duty or obligation to perform a particular service and/or provide care to an individual.
2. There was a breach of this duty that fell below the applicable standard of care.
3. There was a proximate cause that links the breach of this duty directly to the injury being alleged by the plaintiff.
4. There was an injury to the individual that occurred as a result of the breach of duty.

Despite the obvious onset of an acute delirium, brought on by the use of two centrally acting medications (Ativan and Buspar) with drug-drug interaction potential, the nursing home allowed this resident to deteriorate literally in front of their eyes. When he became even more confused, they requested and received an order for a medication that could easily contribute to a worsening of his delirium. The signs and symptoms of acute delirium should be well known to all licensed personnel working in the long-term care environment, and they should have insisted that the attending physician see the resident prior to his ordering the antianxiety medication, Ativan, at such a high initial dosage. In fact, the initial confusion seen in this resident just after admission to the nursing home was probably due to the acute change in his usual environment, rather than a psychiatrically related condition.

The decline in food and fluid intake secondary to his increased sedation and confusion would eventually lead to his severe dehydration and ultimately his demise. A significant decline in nutritional intake needs to be taken seriously. Also, consultations that list an acute medical illness (e.g., delirium) need to be brought to the attending physician's attention in a timely fashion. The issues raised in a consultation need to be addressed in a progress note.

CASE # 2*

An 81-year-old African American male was admitted to Holly Manor Nursing Home from the general hospital for chronic care. His past medical history revealed that he was a non-insulin-dependent diabetic, was S/P a left below-the-knee amputation for vascular disease, and was legally blind. At the time of admission the only medication he was taking was Glucotrol 5 mg once a day for control of diabetes. He could ambulate with a left leg prosthesis without difficulty.

Summary of Events

1. Approximately 6 months after admission, the resident's behavior began to change, and he was noted to have fallen multiple times when ambulating. The nursing care plan was never updated to address these two new problems.

2. Three months later (9 months after admission) Glucotrol was stopped by the attending physician, as the resident's blood sugars seemed fairly well controlled by diet alone. A monthly fasting blood sugar (FBS) was ordered for the next 3 months.

3. The three monthly FBS's were never subsequently done, and the attending physician, on monthly rounds, never noticed this omission from the medical record.

4. At the end of this 3-month period (approximately 1 year after admission), the resident developed a fever associated with a significant decrease in appetite and fluid intake, which was duly noted in the nursing notes but not called to the attention of the attending physician. Fevers to 101.0° F were subsequently recorded for 3 consecutive days, but, again, the attending physician was never called with this information. At the end of the third day the evening staff noticed the resident to be relatively unresponsive, and an order was obtained from the covering physician for an ambulance to transfer the resident. The resident subsequently required intubation at the nursing home by the EMT-Ps and was then transported to the local

---

*All names and places have been changed to protect the confidentiality of this case.

TABLE 13.2 Lab Data

Nursing home (4 months earlier)	Glu 107	BUN 17	Cr 0.9	Na 145
Hospital emergency department	Glu 656	BUN 99	Cr 3.9	Na 171
Dx: Hyperosmolar coma				
Severe dehydration				
Sepsis				

hospital emergency department. The patient died several days after an ICU admission despite multiple interventions. A malpractice suit was subsequently instituted against the nursing home. (See Table 13.2 for a review of laboratory data for both the LTC facility and the hospital.)

Discussion Questions

1. Does the estate of the plaintiff have a real complaint against the nursing home?
2. Should the attending physician have been named as an additional defendant in the suit?
3. Where did the attending physician fail to act properly?
4. Where did the nursing home fail to intervene properly?
5. Could this legal action have been avoided?

Comments

There were many errors made in the management of this resident that contributed to his demise. The change in behavior and falls were never fully evaluated and the nursing care plan was never updated. The FBS tests, which would have detected the loss of diet control of the diabetes, were never drawn. High fevers, which contributed to the development of his severe dehydration, were never called to the attending physician's attention.

Any acute change in mental status or change in functional ability needs to be thoroughly evaluated by the attending physician or his or her designee. Acute medical illness accounts for the vast majority of the reasons such changes are seen in the long-term care environment. Although the attending physician certainly made some clinical errors (e.g., failing to detect the missed FBS results), the plaintiff's attorney felt the majority of the negligence was the nursing home's responsibility. The lawyer believed the staff should have been more diligent in alerting the attending physician to the change in mental status, the febrile episodes, and the decrease in food and fluid intake during the week prior to the resident's acute hospitalization. This case was eventually settled out of court for $500,000.

Multiple-Choice Questions

1. All of the following are possible causes of increased risk for residents except:

A. Failure of the covering physician to return nursing home inquiries.
B. Failure of staff to report serious changes in a resident's condition in the middle of the night to the attending physician.
C. Increased monitoring of a resident with changes from baseline functional status.
D. Failure to document changes in a resident's condition in the medical record.

2. All of the following are methods of establishing a risk management program in a long-term care facility except:

A. Establish a risk management committee.
B. Refer all complaints from families to the facility's attorney immediately.
C. Offer regular in-service presentations on risk management issues.
D. Actively involve the medical director in all risk management programs.

3. All of the following are actions by nursing home staff or attending physicians to maintain a positive medical record except:

A. Avoiding criticizing other staff in the medical record.
B. Avoiding writing damaging comments in the record that have no factual basis.
C. Changing medical orders just to "get back" at "meddling regulations."
D. Documenting the response to ordered medical treatments, even if the response is very poor.

4. In general, the basis for most problems involving lawsuits against nursing homes involves:

A. A desire by the attorney for economic gain.
B. The family's wish to have their name in the newspapers.
C. Poor communication between staff and family members regarding a resident's medical condition or care.
D. Declining number of lawsuits involving acute care hospitals.

5. *Usual targets of discovery in any lawsuit include all of the following* <u>except</u>:

A. Salary records of staff.
B. Medical and nursing notes.
C. Resident care plans.
D. Medication administration sheets.

Answers

1. C
2. B
3. C
4. C
5. A

Resources

Additional resources for information on risk management and other related topics in long-term care may be obtained from the following organizations/sources:

ELDER ABUSE/NEGLECT

The Early Recognition of Elder Abuse: A Quick Reference Guide
Available from American Medical Publishing Co. Inc.
P.O. Box 604885
Bayside, NY 11360
(800) 263-3782

National Center on Elder Abuse
c/o American Public Welfare Association
810 First St. NE, Suite 500
Washington, DC 20002
(202) 682-2470

National Committee for the Prevention of Elder Abuse
c/o Institute on Aging, Medical Center of Central Massachusetts
111 Belmont St.
Worcester, MA 01605
(508) 793-6166

MEDICAL DIRECTION

American Geriatrics Society
770 Lexington Ave., Suite 300
New York, NY 10021
(212) 308-1414
Available: Variety of educational and policy materials on geriatric-related topics.

Medical Direction in the Nursing Home: Principles and Concepts for Physician Administrators
James J. Pattee, M.D.
North Ridge Press
5500 Boone Ave. N.
Minneapolis, MN 55428

RISK MANAGEMENT/ACCREDITATION

ECRI (a nonprofit agency)
Publishers of: *Issues in Continuing Care Risk Management*
5200 Butler Pike
Plymouth Meeting, PA 19462
(610) 825-6000

Joint Commission on Accreditation of Healthcare Organizations
1 Renaissance Blvd.
Oakbrook Terrace, IL 60181
(708) 966-5600
Publishers of: *Accreditation Manual for Long Term Care*
              Standards and Survey Protocols for Dementia Special Care Units

SAFETY ISSUES

American Medical Association
515 North State St.
Chicago, IL 60610
(800) 621-8335
Available: Guidelines on the use of restraints in long-term care facilities.

Occupational Safety and Health Administration (OSHA)
U.S. Department of Labor
Office of Information and Consumer Affairs
200 Constitution Ave., NW
Room N3647
Washington, DC 20210
(202) 219-8151

Untie the Elderly®
The Kendal Corporation
P.O. Box 100
Kennett Square, PA 19348
Available: Resource manuals and videotapes on reducing restraints

TRAINING PROGRAMS

American Health Care Association
Publications Department B1
P.O. Box 96906
Washington, DC 20090
Available: Multitude of training materials/programs on restraint reduction and
   other topics.

Appendix A
Model Set of Bylaws

The quality of medical care in this facility is the responsibility of the Governing Body, the Active Organized Medical Board, and the attending medical staff. These parties hereby agree to adopt the following set of bylaws, regulations, and rules in order to properly discharge that responsibility.

ARTICLE I

A. To ensure that all residents admitted to this facility or treated here receive the best possible care.
B. To provide a means of communication between the medical staff, the Governing Body, and the administration.
C. To initiate and maintain rules and regulations for the government of the medical staff, both Active Organized and the other attending staff.

ARTICLE II

A. Qualifications

All members of the medical staff shall be graduates of an approved or recognized medical or osteopathic school. Members shall possess a full and unrestricted license to practice medicine in the state. Members shall fulfill the requirements for membership on the staff of a general hospital. Physician assistants and nurse practitioners working under the direct supervision of an attending physician in this facility shall meet all state licensing and educational requirements and shall have their scope of practice defined by applicable state regulations and their supervising physician.

B. Ethics

The principles of medical ethics as adopted or amended by the county, State Medical Association, or the state legislature shall govern the professional conduct of a member of the Medical Staff.

C. Composition

The attending medical staff of this facility shall include the Organized Medical Board and the attending staff. The attending staff is comprised of physicians and those nurse practitioners and physician assistants working under the direct supervision of their respective physicians.

D. Organized Medical Board

1. General

The Organized Medical Board membership is drawn from the attending medical staff. In its deliberations, the Organized Medical Board is assisted by the Director of Nursing Services (an RN) and the Executive Director/Administrator. These last two named positions have the responsibility of furnishing the physicians with data and appropriate details regarding each patient's care requirements as well as up-to-date details on Medicare and Medicaid regulations. Other nonphysician members may include representatives from other departments at the facility. Consultations may be requested from other individuals, including consulting psychiatrists, dentists, podiatrists, pharmacists, physical therapists, dietitians, social workers, and medical records personnel.

2. Members and Officers

The Organized Medical Board shall consist of at least three physicians from the attending medical staff. A chairman shall be nominated and elected by the membership at the annual meeting and shall serve for a period of one year. Members will be chosen regardless of sex, race, creed, color, or sexual preferences. The Medical Director may serve as chairman.

3. Object of the Organized Medical Board

The function of the Organized Medical Board shall be to act in an advisory capacity in the planning of all policies concerning medical matters in order to achieve and maintain high standards of patient care.

4. Meetings

Regular meetings will be held every ninety (90) days. The annual meeting will be held at the discretion of the committee. Time and place of the meetings may be held at the discretion of the Executive Director after consultation with the Chairman. The meeting is called to order by the Chairman and the members will review the minutes of the previous meeting.

5. Requirements of Members

  a. Members of the Organized Medical Board shall be required to attend at least fifty percent (50%) of the medical staff meetings.
  b. The Organized Medical Board shall adopt written bylaws governing the medical care of the facility's patients. Such bylaws shall be approved by the Medical Director and the Governing Body. The bylaws shall be developed so as to direct all areas of patient care and treatment in the facility. In addition, these bylaws shall include standards of practice, verification of credentials, privileging, etc., as well as specify the duties of the Medical Director and Governing Body to enforce these standards.
  c. Upon appointment to the Attending Medical Staff, each member shall sign the bylaws and be governed accordingly.

E. Attending Medical Staff

1. General

  The attending medical staff shall consist of those physicians who are permitted privileges to admit and treat residents at this facility. Privileges will be extended to those physicians determined through mutual agreement by the Executive Director, the Medical Director, and the Organized Medical Board.

2. Requirements of the Attending Medical Staff

  a. Members of the attending medical staff shall satisfy the specific standards and criteria set in these medical bylaws of the facility.
  b. Members shall be available by telephone twenty-four (24) hours per day and be available to respond promptly in an emergency, and be able to provide an alternate physician for coverage whenever necessary.
  c. Members shall maintain adequate medical malpractice liability insurance.
  d. Upon application to the attending medical staff, the physician shall acquaint himself/herself with the bylaws, rules, and regulations of the facility and attest to his/her agreement in writing.
  e. Members shall annually supply a copy of their license, malpractice insurance, and hospital affiliation and agree to the bylaws, rules, and regulations of the facility.

3. Terms of Appointment

  a. The Medical Director and Executive Director shall approve or deny applications for membership on the Organized Medical Board and attending staff after consultation with the existing Organized Medical Board, if any, and subject to the ratification of the Governing Body. In reviewing the applicant, the Medical Director shall consider the applicant's ability to meet the criteria and standards set forth in these regulations. The Medical Director may grant temporary privileges to a physician subject to review at the next scheduled meeting of the Organized Medical Board.

b. All appointments shall be made in writing and shall delineate the physician's duties and responsibilities. The letter of appointment shall be signed by the Medical Director, the Executive Director, and the applicant.

c. Appointments shall be for the period of the calendar year. Reappointment shall be made for two (2) years at the start of the calendar year.

ARTICLE III

A. Standards of Practice

1. All patients/residents at (name of facility) shall be promptly admitted to this facility by the attending physician in accordance with the facility policies governing admission and with respect to the State and Federal Regulations governing admission.

2. All patients/residents will, annually, receive a comprehensive physical examination by their attending physician, or designated health care provider (e.g., physician assistant or nurse practitioner).

3. Specific laboratory, visual, and auditory testing as well as permissible immunization will be performed within the time frames as established by this state. These will be in addition to any testing which may be periodically required because of condition, medication, or other factors necessitating such testing. Physicians may also order specific testing as necessary. No testing or immunizations will be performed if they are medically contraindicated or if the patient or their conservator refuse and any such refusal shall be properly documented in the medical record.

4. The Medical Director shall review specific cases at the request of the Director of Nursing under the following circumstances:

a. The patient/resident's attending physician is unable or unwilling to be of assistance and the patient/resident's condition appears to warrant immediate attention.

b. The patient/resident is requesting admission and based on information provided, a question as to the appropriateness of placement or the facility's ability to care for the person arises. Under these conditions, the Medical Director shall be fully advised of the situation and the facility will abide by his/her decision to either approve or deny admission.

5. Summaries of previous medical treatments will be obtained from the persons or facilities providing the services.

6. Active patient care planning involving all departments will commence on admission and continue for the duration of the patient's stay in the facility. Such planning will be done in accordance with the time frames established by this state but may be done more frequently if needed.

7. Adequate information will be provided at the time of discharge or transfer to the receiving facility in order to provide proper care and treatment of the patient/resident. Such information will contain at least the specifics stated in the Public Health Code as well as any additional information which may aid in caring for the patient.

8. Physicians, physician assistants, and nurse practitioners admitting residents shall be held responsible for giving such information as may be necessary to assure the protection of other residents from those who are a source of danger from any cause whatever or to assure protection of the resident from self-harm.

9. All orders for treatment shall be in writing. An order shall be considered to be in writing if dictated to a nurse registered in this state and signed by the attending physician within the required time frame. Orders dictated over the telephone shall be signed by the nurse to whom dictated, with the name of the physician, physician assistant, or nurse practitioner. The attending physician shall sign orders within the required time frame.

10. Narcotics may be prescribed for within the guidelines as established by this facility's policies. Physician assistants or nurse practitioners may only write for narcotic medications as permitted under the laws of this state. Drugs used shall be those listed in the U.S. Pharmacopedia, National Formulary, New and Non-Official Remedies, with the exception of drugs for bona fide clinical investigations.

11. The attending physician, physician assistant, or nurse practitioner shall be held responsible for the preparation of a complete medical record for each resident in accordance with State Code and requirement found in the Medical and Professional Service Policies. This record shall include:

    a. Admission history and physical examination

    b. Progress notes

    c. Written medical orders

12. No medical record shall be filed until it is complete, except on order of the Medical Records Committee. The charts of all residents who have died must be completed within thirty (30) days.

13. All records are the property of the long-term care facility and shall not be taken away without permission. In case of the readmission of a resident, all previous records shall be available for the use of the attending physician, physician assistant, or nurse practitioner.

14. Each member of the medical staff shall name qualified alternates who may be called to attend a resident in the event that he/she is not available. In case of failure to name such a member, the Executive Director of the facility shall have the authority to call the Medical Director who will provide services to the resident as needed.

15. Residents shall be discharged only on orders of the attending physician or against medical advice should the physician not give an order for discharge. At the time of discharge the attending physician shall write his/her discharge diagnosis and sign the record. Records shall be completed within thirty (30) days after discharge.

16. If autopsies are desirable and efforts are made to obtain them, written consent of next of kin must be obtained. All autopsies must be performed by a qualified pathologist.

17. Members of the medical staff shall request medical consultations when indications exist of an obscure diagnosis/problem or when there is doubt as to the treatment. The consultant shall be qualified in the field in which the opinion is sought and the consultation shall include examination of the patient and medical records.

B. Medical Director

1. The Medical Director shall be a physician licensed to practice medicine in this state and shall serve on the facility's Organized Medical Board, shall have at least one (1) year prior clinical experience in adult medicine, and shall be a member of the active medical staff of a general hospital licensed in this state.

2. The Medical Director shall have the following powers and responsibilities:

    a. Enforce the facility's bylaws governing medical care.

    b. Assure that quality medical care is provided in this state.

    c. Serve as liaison between the medical staff and administration.

    d. Approve or disapprove a patient's admission based on the facility's ability to provide adequate care for that individual in accordance with the facility's bylaws. The Medical Director shall have the authority to review any patient's record or examine any patient prior to admission for that purpose.

    e. Assure that each patient in the facility has an assigned personal physician.

    f. Provide or arrange for the provision of necessary medical care to the patient if the individual's personal physician is unable or unwilling to do so.

    g. Approve or deny applications for membership of the facility's medical staff.

    h. In accordance with the facility's bylaws, suspend or terminate the facility privileges of a medical staff member if that member is unable or unwilling to adequately care for a patient in accordance with standards set by any applicable local and state statutes and regulations, any federal regulations that may apply to a federal program in which the facility participates, or facility bylaws.

i. Visit the facility within the hours of 7:00 A.M. and 9:00 P.M. to assess the adequacy of medical care provided in the facility at least once every seven (7) days.

j. Receive reports from the Director of Nursing on significant clinical developments.

k. Recommend to the Executive Director any purchases of medical equipment and/or services necessary to assure adequate patient care.

l. Assist in the development of and participate in a staff orientation and training program in cooperation with the Executive Director and the Director of Nursing.

m. A record shall be kept by the facility of the Medical Director's visits and statements for review by the Department. Such record shall minimally include the date of visit and a summary of problems discussed with the staff.

n. Participate in staff meetings which include, but are not limited to, Medical Staff, Infection Control, Pharmaceutical Services, CQI, Patient Care Policies, and advise the Admission and Staff Education committees.

o. Implement methods that assure surveillance of the health status of employees, including routine health examinations and freedom from infections.

p. Recommend and participate in the educational programs of the facility.

ARTICLE IV

A. Amendments

1. Amendments or revisions of these bylaws may be made by the Organized Medical Board. Any amendment or revision must be circulated to the full Organized Medical Board at least two (2) weeks prior to a regularly scheduled meeting. A majority vote of those present at that meeting shall be sufficient to amend or revise these bylaws.

ARTICLE V

A. Disciplinary Action of Member of Medical Staff

1. The Medical Director and Executive Director of this facility shall grant or deny privileges to physicians interested in attending residents at this facility in accordance with medical board bylaws.

2. The Medical Director is also charged with the responsibility of taking any disciplinary action that may be required against those physicians who presently are on staff.

3. Suspension of privileges or other disciplinary measures shall be initiated by the Medical Director if the physician in question in his/her opinion is jeopardizing the delivery of good resident care to his/her residents at (name of facility).

4. Disciplinary action may result from noncompliance with applicable State and Federal regulations governing physician services.

B. Suspension of Privileges

1. The suspension of medical privileges may result if the physician in question:

a. Does not conform to State and Federal regulations after having received two (2) formal requests (letters from Medical Director and/or Executive Director).

b. Exhibits gross negligence or incompetence in dispensing medical care to his/her residents at this facility. In this case, the Medical Director, if he/she deems it appropriate and necessary, may suspend said privileges immediately.

c. The Organized Medical Board shall approve all actions of the Medical Director at the next regularly scheduled meeting, or sooner at the call of the Medical Director.

2. Should a physician either receive some form of disciplinary action or be suspended and wish to contest the action, he/she may proceed with Procedure I or Procedure II.

C. Due Process of Appeal

1. Procedure I

a. Request the Executive Director to place him on the agenda for the next regularly scheduled Organized Medical Board committee meeting.

b. Present his/her position before the Organized Medical Board committee meeting, citing specific reasons why the action taken was unfair, inappropriate, or too severe.

c. Request the Organized Medical Board committee lift any and all sanctions or modify such sanctions.

d. The Organized Medical Board committee shall, with a majority vote, rule on said request with its decision binding.

e. In the event that a physician had admitting privileges suspended indefinitely and said suspension was upheld by the Organized Medical Board, the physician may reapply for admitting privileges in twelve (12) months following the above action.

2. Procedure II
   a. Request a hearing panel consisting of three (3) members as follows:
      i. A licensed physician attending one or more residents at this facility to be appointed by the Medical Director.
      ii. A licensed physician attending one or more residents at this facility to be appointed by the aggrieved physician.
      iii. A licensed physician attending one or more residents at this facility (and mutually agreeable to the appointment by both the Medical Director and the aggrieved physician) shall be the third member of the panel.
   b. The aggrieved physician shall:
      i. Present his/her position before the three (3) member panel and cite specific reasons why the action taken was unfair, inappropriate, or too severe.
      ii. Request the three (3) member panel lift any and all sanctions or to modify such sanctions.
   c. The three (3) member panel shall, with a majority vote, rule on said request with its decision binding on the Organized Medical Board committee and on the aggrieved physician.
   d. In the event that a physician had admitting privileges suspended indefinitely and said suspension was upheld by the three (3) member panel, the physician may reapply for admitting privileges in twelve (12) months following the above action.

RULES AND REGULATIONS

Medical and Professional Services

Supervision of Medical Care

The medical care of this facility is under the direct supervision of the Medical Director, who is a licensed physician in this state and who participates in planning and organizing the medical care of this facility. The Medical Director assists in developing established policies and procedures of this facility and reviews them at least annually.

A. A comprehensive history and medical examination shall be completed for each patient within forty-eight (48) hours of admission; however, if the physician who attended the patient in an acute or chronic care hospital is the same physician who will attend the individual in the facility, a copy of a hospital discharge summary completed within five (5) working days of admission and accompanying the patient may serve in lieu of this requirement. A patient assessment and patient care plan shall be developed within seven (7) days of admission.

1. The comprehensive history shall include, but not be limited to:

   a. Chief complaints
   b. History of present illness
   c. Review of systems
   d. Past history pertinent to the total plan of care for the patient
   e. Family medical history pertinent to the total plan of care for the patient
   f. Personal and social history
   g. Functional status
   h. Advance Directives

2. The comprehensive examination shall include, but not be limited to:

   a. Vital signs, including pulse and blood pressure
   b. Weight
   c. Physical exam findings as noted on the admission examination form
   d. Rectal examination with a test for occult blood in stool, unless done within one (1) year of admission

B. Transferred Patients

   When the responsibility for the care of a patient is being transferred from one health care institution to another, the patient must be accompanied by a medical information transfer document, which shall include the following information:

1. Chief complaints, problems, or diagnosis
2. Other information, including physical or mental limitation, allergies, behavioral and management problems
3. Any special diet requirements
4. Any current medications or treatments

C. The attending physician shall record a summary of findings, problems, and diagnosis based on the data available within forty-eight (48) hours after the patient's admission including, but not limited to, an overall treatment plan, dietary orders and rehabilitation potential, and, if indicated, further laboratory, radiological, or other testing, consultations, medications and other treatment, and limitations on activities.

D. The tests and procedures shall be performed as ordered by the attending physician.

E. At the time of each visit the attending physician renews and/or revises his/her patient's total program of care, which includes, but is not limited to, physician orders for medications, treatments, rehabilitative nursing, physical therapy treatment, diet, and precautions related to activities undertaken by the patient; the physician records his/her visits and progress notes.

F. No medication or treatments shall be given without a physician's order. If orders are given verbally or by telephone, they shall be recorded by a licensed nurse on duty with a physician's name and shall be signed by the physician within the required time frame.

G. Annually, each patient shall receive a comprehensive medical examination, at which time the attending physician, or designated health care provider, shall update the diagnosis and revise the individual's overall treatment plan in accordance with such diagnosis. The comprehensive medical exam shall minimally include those services required as stated in a previous section of this document. The annual medical examination is dated and signed by the physician or designee.

H. Restraints: Use of restraints will be per this facility's guidelines and policies.

I. The requirements in this sections for tests, procedures, and immunizations need not be repeated if previously done within the usual time period and documentation of such is recorded in the patient's medical record. Such tests, procedures, and immunizations shall be provided to the patient given the individual's consent provided no medical reason or contraindication exists.

J. In the even of the death of a patient/resident, the attending physician shall:

1. Personally pronounce the patient's death, unless an order for nurse pronouncement is in place.
2. Complete a Death Certificate, discharge summary, and progress note detailing the time and cause of death.
3. Notify the patient/resident's family.
4. When required, notify the Medical Examiner.
5. Give orders regarding the disposition of the deceased.

Medical Emergencies

A. Care of Residents in Emergencies

In the event of a medical emergency to an individual or individuals, first aid treatment is rendered under the direction of the attending physician. If the attending physician is unavailable, the covering physician will be contacted. If neither physician is available, the Medical Director or his/her designee will be contacted and informed as to the emergency and appropriate measures taken. When ordered by the physician, the resident will be transferred to the Emergency Room of the nearest general hospital for further treatment.

B. Communicable Disease Outbreak:

1. All communicable diseases will be reviewed by the Infection Control Committee and necessary measures will be taken according to their policies.
2. If there is a sufficient number of communicable diseased residents, then the residents will be isolated to a specific area to prevent further outbreak of the disease. The remaining residents and visitors will be restricted from this area unless specified by the Infection Control Committee. Specific isolation techniques will be instituted by all personnel.

C. Critically Ill Residents:

1. When there is a change in the resident's condition, the attending physician or nurse in charge, under the direction of the attending physician, will notify the family concerning the change. The resident and/or family will be consulted as to the choice of treatment.
2. Documentation in the medical record is necessary if the resident and/or family refuses further medical treatment.

D. Mentally Disturbed Residents:

1. If a resident becomes disturbed and unmanageable while at this facility, orders for restraints or sedating medications should be obtained from the attending physician.
2. If a resident remains disturbed and unmanageable, the physician will be notified regarding transfer to the appropriate facility.

Director of Nursing Communications to the Medical Director Regarding Significant Clinical Developments

The Director of Nursing will discuss significant clinical developments with the Supervising Physician on a weekly basis (or more frequently, as needed). The

Supervising Physician will in turn communicate these clinical issues to the Medical Director as well as any orders/interventions that have been prescribed if the clinical situation warrants such communication. Appropriate documentation will be included on the chart and daily rounds sheet. If the Supervising Physician or his/her covering physician is not available at the time a significant clinical development occurs, the DNS will contact the Medical Director by phone and document this conversation on the clinical observation record.

Appendix B

Model Application for Clinical Privileges

APPLICATION FOR CLINICAL PRIVILEGES FOR MEDICAL SERVICE

Name: _____Degree: _____

I am applying for privileges to perform the following services or procedures for which I am qualified by training and experience:

( )   General medical coverage of nursing home residents, including the differential diagnosis and treatment of common geriatric syndromes

( )   Consultation privileges only in the field of _____(specify)

( )   Other procedures to be performed in the nursing home setting (specify)

_____

_____

I agree to furnish with this request a Xerox copy of my:

• State medical license
• Federal DEA reg. # (if applicable)
• State narcotic reg. # (if applicable)
• Proof of malpractice insurance
• Proof of hospital staff membership or a written statement documenting that I have no current membership

Signature of provider requesting privileges: _____
Date: /   /

Approved: _____ Medical Director
          (on behalf of the Medical Board of XYZ Nursing Center)   Date: /   /

Approved: _____ Administrator
          (on behalf of the XYZ Nursing Center)   Date: /   /

Facility Use Only:

Name of applicant requesting privileges: _____

Privileges requested: _____ Date application received: /   /

Credentialing Information Received:
Copy of:
[   ] State license   Date received: /   /
[   ] Federal DEA reg. #   Date received: /   /
[   ] State narcotic reg. # (if applicable)   Date received: /   /
[   ] Proof of malpractice insurance   Date received: /   /
[   ] Proof of hospital staff membership   Date received: /   /
      - OR -
[   ] State Medical Society credential check Date received: /   /

1) Date reviewed by Medical Director/Medical Board: /   /

Action taken by Medical Board: Approved   Disapproved

2) Date reviewed by Administrator: /   /

Action taken by Administrator: Approved   Disapproved

3) Date applicant notified by facility: /   /

COMMENTS:
_____
_____

Index

Abuse
  documentation of, 38t
  intervention strategies for, 41t–42t
  investigation of, 36–37
    protocol, 39f–41f
  legal aspects of, 60
  major indicators of, 36, 36t
  prevention of, 35–43
  reporting, 76
  resources on, 95
  sexual, signs of, 37
  taking seriously, 79
Accreditation by JCAHO, 55
  resources on, 96
Acute illness, spread of, 32–33
Administration, active participation of, 4
Admissions, new. *See* New admissions
Affidavit, sample, 64–68
Air changes per hour, for isolation rooms,
  30
Alprazolam, dosage for, 26t
American Medical Director's Association
  (AMDA), 53
  policy on role of medical director,
    54f–55f
Analgesics, side effects of, 24t
Anticholinergic medications, side effects
  of, 24t
Antiemetics, side effects of, 24t
Antihistamines
  falls caused by, 49t
  side effects of, 24t
Anti-Parkinsonian drugs, falls caused by,
  49t
Antipsychotic drugs
  counterindications for, 24
  side effects of, 24t

Antiseizure drugs, falls caused by, 49t
Antispasmodics, side effects of, 24t
Anxiolytic agents, dosage for, 26t
Application for clinical privileges, model
  of, 113–114
Assault, resident against resident, 46–48
  legal aspects of, 60
Atarax, dosage for, 26t
Ativan, dosage for, 26t
Attitude, positive, importance of, 77
Audience, for risk management guide, 2

Behavioral concerns, and medication,
  14–15
Benadryl, side effects of, 24t
Benzodiazepines
  falls caused by, 49t
  limitations of, 25–26
  side effects of, 24t
Bleeding, response required for, 74t
Burnout, prevention of, 37–38
BuSpar, dosage for, 26t
Buspirone HCL, dosage for, 26t
Bylaws for staff, 53–55, 99–111

Carisoprodol, side effects of, 24t
C. difficile infections, control policy, 31
Chest pain, response required for, 74t
Chloral hydrate, dosage for, 26t
Clinical privileges, model application for,
  113–114
Communication
  about medication, 15
  importance of, 2, 4, 84
Computers, training in, 72–73
Consent, informed, 35, 60
Contingency plans, 6

Problems
  following up on, 63
  procedure for response to, 77
  staff review of, 56
Progress notes, maintenance of, 76
Propoxyphene, side effects of, 24t
Psychotropic drugs, falls caused by, 49t
Punishment, corporal, 35

Quality control, 4

Rashes, response required for, 74t
Recommendations
  for isolation room air changes, 30
  for risk management, 77–79
Records, maintenance of, 73t
Residents
  assault by, 46–48, 60
  elopement risks, 60
  legal rights of, 35
  missing, protocol for location of, 47t
  pre-admission evaluation of, 57, 85
Respirators, TB, CDC recommendation
  for, 30
Restraints, 20–21, 35
  alternatives to, 20–21
  committee on, 78
  danger of, 20, 22t
  definition of, 20
  FDA recommendations for, 23t
  legal requirements for, 21
Retraining, importance of, 6
Review, pre-admission, 57, 85
Risk management
  areas of concern, 1, 5
  committee for, 77–78
  definition of, 1
  future of, 84–86
  implementation of program, 71–83
  key areas of, 3–4
  legal aspects of, 60–70
  recommendations for, 77–79
  resources on, 96
  team, formation of, 4
Robaxin, side effects of, 24t

Safe Medical Devices Act of 1990, 21
Safety, 44–52
  resources on, 96–97
Seclusion, involuntary, 35
Sedative-hypnotics, side effects of, 24t

Sedatives, falls caused by, 49t
Seizures, response required for, 74t
Serax, dosage for, 26t
Sexual abuse, signs of, 37
Shortness of breath, response required for,
  74t
Skin care team, 78–79
Smoking, 49–50
Soma, side effects of, 24t
Staff
  bylaws for, 53–55, 99–111
  communication with medical director,
    55–58, 62
  exploitation by plaintiff, 63
  health of, 55f
  privileges of, 55–56
  proper training of, 6, 63
  workplace risk factors, 50–51
Subacute units, 5–6

TB. See Tuberculosis
Tigan, side effects of, 24t
Training, in-service, 4, 76
  in computers, 72–73
  documentation of, 6, 73
  importance of, 84
  and medication, 15, 26–27
  refreshing of, 6
  resources on, 97
Trimethobenzamide, side effects of, 24t
Tuberculosis, infection control policy,
  29–30
  filtering masks, 30
  in-service education on, 30

Ulcers. See Pressure ulcers
42 U.S.C. 1396r (1990 sup.), 61

Vaccine programs, 31
Vistaril, dosage for, 26t
Vital signs, changes in, response required
  for, 74t
VREF infections, control policy, 31

Wandering, 44–46. See also Elopement
  dangers of, 46
  legal aspects of, 60
  management of, 45–46, 47t
  types of, 45
Workplace risk factors, 50–51

Xanax, dosage for, 26t